LIVE FIT AND BE WELL
A Personal Transformation Workbook

Erik Hajer

Hajer House Publishing · Newton, Massachusetts

Disclaimer

Live Fit and Be Well: A Personal Transformation Workbook is intended for healthy adults age 18 and older. It is solely for informational and educational purposes and are not intended for medical advice. Please consult a medical or health professional before starting any new exercise, nutrition, or wellness program or if you have questions about your health. To protect their identity, the names of individuals featured in *Live Fit and Be Well* have been changed.

This workbook is dedicated to all the extraordinary people
I have had the privilege to coach with over the last sixteen years.
It's through our journey together that this book was born.
Therefore, it's as much your creation as it is mine.

Table of Contents and Chapter Synopses

Synopsis: Part I will help you discover and unleash your personal power by giving you the tools to take consistent, inspired action throughout your life journey. You will also learn how to break through obstacles, such as limiting beliefs, habits, and fears, which may have derailed you in the past.

Part II: Breakthrough Fitness System

Synopsis: Part II invites you to make your breakthrough fitness connection for life with a transformative 90-day jumpstart fitness program. The intention of the Breakthrough Fitness System is to help you create a personal exercise program that is fun, effective, and fits into the fabric of your life. To help you do this, I've developed a system that you can do at your health club as well as an express circuit that requires no added equipment and can be done in the comfort of your home. This unique system combines the fundamentals of exercise science with leading-edge training techniques, such as interval training, dynamic weight training, plyometrics, anaerobic threshold training, functional training, Pilates, and yoga.

Part III: Mindful Eating

Synopsis: Mindful Eating empowers you to enjoy all that food has to offer while nourishing, healing, and energizing your body and your life. Part III invites you to discover an intuitive way of eating that supports abundant health and wellness and does not require obsessive dieting, deprivation, or "willpower."

Part IV: Living Wellness ....

Synopsis: In Part IV you will learn how nurturing your whole life can have an immediate impact on your health and your ability to take consistent, inspired action. You will explore how your wellness is tied not only to how you eat, move, and think, but also to your relationships, work environment, responsibilities, and more. Part IV invites you to unite your plan by offering strategies for staying on your fitness and wellness path for life.

An Invitation

There are many reasons you may have decided to start a fitness and wellness program. You may be feeling frustrated, out of shape, and stuck in a body that's holding you back from the life you want to live. You may be tired of quick-fix diet and exercise programs. You may be looking for a new way of doing things—a plan that breaks you of your old patterns and beliefs. Or you may have hit a plateau after training successfully for years. No matter what your past story, making the decision to evolve from wherever you are now is a powerful first step. So let me take this opportunity to formally invite you to discover your true potential and start living the extraordinary life you deserve.

My name is Erik Hajer, known to many as Coach E, and I want to thank you for giving me the opportunity to be your partner on your fitness and wellness journey. For the record, I am *not* another diet and exercise sage. I created this workbook with the belief that you hold the master key to your own transformation. You are creative, resourceful, and brilliant! You may have been derailed in the past, but, no matter what, you can overcome any obstacles that try to stand in your way. The reason is, the power you need does not lie somewhere "out there" but *within you.*

This workbook is about giving you the tools to awaken your power to make *your* lasting fitness and wellness connections. It's about creating a mindset and lifestyle that support living well. And it's about thriving as opposed to just surviving.

You deserve to feel more than just "fine." You deserve to feel fantastic. You deserve to live your dreams! With that intention, I invite you to join me in a partnership. I cannot climb the mountain for you; however, I can be your guide, help you find *your* path, and support you every step of the way. If you're ready to live as the fit, vital, and empowered person you can and deserve to be, then together we can do what may have once seemed impossible.

> " *Change is often a result of lighting a fire under you. Lasting transformation is a result of lighting a fire within you! —Coach E*

Make Your Connection

We've been taught to believe that if we want to change our bodies, we must focus exclusively on diet and exercise. This belief is fueled by the notion that the body is a problem that needs to be fixed. And the measuring stick of success is often an unrealistic, "ideal" body that has been determined by popular culture, advertising, and quick-fix diet plans and drugs. Plugging into this ideal is like building a house without a foundation. The frame may sustain itself over a brief period of time, but a house without a strong foundation will eventually collapse.

Following a plan that prescribes strict diet and exercise rules eventually causes most people to rebel and give up. No wonder so many people have difficulty staying on track with traditional plans! Imagine, instead, how it would feel to transform by developing a sustainable and enjoyable *lifestyle* that unlocks your potential. Imagine how it would feel to have explosive energy, abundant vitality, and look fantastic to boot.

What is important to remember is that fitness and wellness are intricately linked. Physical fitness is often defined in terms of strength, agility, balance, flexibility, and endurance. I invite you to think of fitness as more than that. When you feel fit, you love the way you look and you love the way you feel. This feeling of empowerment often spreads throughout your entire life. Also, wellness is more than the absence of disease—it is a state of being well in body *and* mind. When you are well in body and mind, you not only feel strong, energetic, and healthy, you feel capable, positive, and happy. Awakening your mind and body is the first step toward accessing the unlimited power of your whole, integrated self.

This workbook is a call to action designed to inspire the real you to emerge. It is a lifestyle system based on the belief that the "whole you" has the power to create enduring fitness and wellness in your life. This holistic approach is a powerful and potent paradigm shift from the mainstream diet and exercise model that focuses on a one-size-fits-all approach to losing weight. This workbook is not just about losing weight, it is a personal guide to living your whole life to its fullest potential.

My Story

My interest in fitness and wellness is a personal one. Growing up I witnessed my mother struggle with obesity and food addiction. It was heartbreaking to watch her, knowing she was stuck in a body that was holding her back from the life she wanted to live. After many years of yo-yo dieting, my mother discovered a holistic approach to wellness. It was the key to her personal transformation.

My mother's journey inspired me to dedicate my professional career to helping others discover their key to lasting fitness and wellness. In 1995, I founded EH Fitness and Wellness Coaching, a whole-health coaching company.

For many years I contemplated the questions: How can people create more wellness in their lives? What are the keys to lifelong fitness success? And why is it so hard for most people to break through their old patterns?

After much trial and error, as well as personal and professional application, I came to the conclusion that there is a universal block preventing most people from awakening their full potential. Ironically,

I found that this block had nothing to do with food or exercise. Almost every client was engaged in a struggle between his or her own thoughts and actions. While most people believed they wanted to get fit and feel more alive and energetic, their thoughts and actions often contradicted their intentions.

Realizing there were limited resources in the fitness market to help people overcome this challenge, I became driven to develop an interactive workbook that combined a leading-edge fitness program, a holistic approach to food, and an accessible system for taking consistent inspired action. The intention was for people to make personal connections to fitness and wellness, and overcome old beliefs and fears for life. And the results were remarkable! I began witnessing amazing breakthroughs and transformations. Not only were people transforming their bodies, but they were living more vital and empowered lives. I knew I had something valuable to share with the world.

It turns out, however, that in my quest to create a workbook to help my clients, I was the first one to be transformed.

For most of my adolescent and adult life, I poured mega amounts of energy into achieving my physical potential, competing in numerous marathons and Ironman Triathlons around the country. While I looked and felt fit, something was always missing. I constantly strived for the next "hit" of feeling fit and well. I never achieved the sustained level of happiness I believed my physical triumphs would yield.

Working the exercises described in this workbook helped me realize that I am so much more than what my body looks like and what it can be trained to do. In fact, it was never about just transforming my body, it was about transforming how I was thinking, how I was feeling, and how I was acting. It was about transforming my life. This was the catalyst to breaking through my own limiting beliefs, habits, and fears that had been preventing me from thriving and feeling fantastic. This integrated approach has helped me reconnect with the whole me. I now know happiness comes from within, and I can happily achieve as opposed to achieve to be happy. For me, this has opened the door to a new way of being that I never dreamed possible. I have never felt more fit, vital, and whole. This is the feeling of fitness and wellness I want to share with you, wherever you may be on your journey and whatever personal block you may want to overcome.

To date, this system has inspired and empowered people of all ages and athletic abilities to not only transform their bodies and take control of their health, but also rediscover their power to create positive energy, meaning, and happiness in their lives. My clients have been my greatest teachers and a source of abundant inspiration. My sincere motivation is that this workbook acts as your guide as you become the person you can and deserve to be. It doesn't have to be a struggle. *You* are the author of your story. *You* can make it happen! I'm excited and grateful to be an ally on your journey.

Let *your* transformation begin!

" *When you are inspired by some great purpose, some extraordinary project, all of your thoughts break their bonds: Your mind transcends limitations, your consciousness expands in every direction, and you find yourself in a new, great, and wonderful world. Dormant forces, faculties, and talents become alive, and [you] discover yourself to be a greater person by far than you ever dreamed yourself to be. —Patanjali*

How to Use This Workbook

As the title suggests, this is not a one-size-fits-all program. Instead, this workbook provides you with an opportunity to develop a personalized plan that unlocks your potential. The intention is to meet you where you are and help you discover *your* master key to living your most fit, vital, and empowered life. To that end, here are a few suggestions to help guide you:

Part I. Turn Your Mind Into an Ally: Empowerment Provisions for Your Journey

The first section will help you discover your personal power and give you the tools to take consistent, inspired action. You will also learn how to break through any inner obstacles that may have derailed you in the past. Many clients who have come to me feeling "stuck" in their old patterns and beliefs have found it beneficial to spend quality time on this section before starting the fitness and nutrition sections; in essence, laying down the mental foundation before building the house.

Part I is not intended to be read and completed all at once. Rather, this first section should be practiced and integrated over time. To get the most out of this section, I suggest doing no more than one "Your Turn" exercise per day. You may even decide to spend multiple days working on a particular exercise. Once you have laid down the groundwork, you will learn how to develop a daily practice—or "mental workout"—to strengthen your empowerment provisions. If you're not ready to address a given area, simply move on to the next exercise. You can always circle back, "rework," and review places where you feel blocked. You may find this section stirs up a host of thoughts, feelings, and emotions. Some exercises may be inspiring and liberating while others may evoke resistance and bring up challenges you've been struggling with for years. Know that any and all reactions you have are okay, and that simply becoming more aware of these thoughts and feelings can be transformative. Give yourself the time and freedom to notice what comes up for you without forcing or judging. Go at your own pace.

Part II. Breakthrough Fitness System and Part III. Mindful Eating

The fitness and nutrition sections provide you with a simple yet effective exercise and mindful eating program that can be personalized to work for you. The system is based on proven exercise techniques and up-to-date nutritional information. These two sections are framed as a 90-day jumpstart program intended to inspire you for a lifetime.

Part IV. Living Wellness

The final section offers you suggestions for staying motivated while leading a happier, healthier, and more vital life. Many clients have found that reading this section while working on their fitness and nutrition plan helps solidify important strategies in connecting physical fitness with overall well-being. For many, this has been a catalyst to breaking through for good.

Remember, *you* hold the master key to your transformation. You may find that some of the exercises, ideas, and suggestions connect with you while others do not. Keep in mind that every sentence in this book is an invitation to discover your own answers. I believe that this is the most powerful way to inspire you to create lasting, lifelong fitness and wellness.

Part I
Turn Your Mind Into an Ally:
Empowerment Provisions for Your Journey

" The real power to transform comes from within. By recognizing and cultivating this power, you awaken your ability to create lasting fitness and wellness in your life. —Coach E

Have you ever felt as if you were fighting your mind as you pursued positive changes in your life? Have you ever felt out of control, behaving in ways you knew did not support your wellness? If so, you are not alone. At one time or another, most of us have experienced self-sabotaging behavior. And we generally rely on willpower to get back on track. However, in most cases, willpower eventually gives way to old habits and behaviors. Without realizing it, we often set ourselves up to fail.

Using willpower to overcome internal roadblocks is like trying to break through an iceberg by chipping away at its tip. Unless you address what lies beneath the surface, you will remain stuck in your old ways. That's because when you rely on willpower to make changes in your life, you are most likely focusing your attention on what you *don't* want. If you're constantly saying, "I don't want to be overweight," you are attracting fear and anxiety about things that contribute to being overweight. Trying to resist what you don't want will only attract more of the same. Whatever you resist, you empower. The transformation begins when you shift your focus from what you don't want to what you do want. For example, "I want to be happy, healthy, and active!"

While most mainstream diet and exercise programs focus on willpower, I invite you to rediscover your "whole power." You'll begin to leverage your whole power when you learn to align your thoughts and actions with what you intend to create in your life. When you unleash your whole power in the direction of your dreams, you become inspired to take action—not because you should but because you *must*. The difference is feeling as if you're purposefully gliding down the river of your life versus forever fighting the current.

To help you cultivate your whole power for your transformation journey, I've created what I call Whole Power Provisions (WPP's). These WPP's are designed to help you take consistent, inspired action, as well as help you overcome any roadblocks that may challenge you along the way.

> " *The moment one definitely commits oneself, then Providence moves too. A whole stream of events issues from the decision, raising in one's favor all manner of unforeseen incidents and meetings and material assistance, which no man could have dreamt would have come his way.*
> —W.H. Murray

I define intention as a clear decision aligned with an inspiring purpose. Living with intention moves you from wanting and hoping to deciding and acting. It allows you to send a clear message to the universe that you are ready to make things happen!

Goal Setting on a Deeper Level

Goal setting is often used to target a desired outcome. When we set goals, we link success and happiness to the end result. What is often forgotten is the purpose for setting the goal, the present and future benefits of working toward the goal, and the joy that can be found along the way.

In his groundbreaking book *Happier*, Tal Ben-Shahar writes, "Happiness is not about making it to the peak of the mountain nor is it about climbing aimlessly around the mountain; happiness is the experience of climbing toward the peak." Happiness is not an end result but the ongoing expression of joy while you evolve and grow.

When I was in high school, I believed that if I made the varsity basketball team, I would be happy and content. I did and I was . . . for a short time. In college, I believed if I radically reduced my body fat and achieved a ripped, muscular look, I would be happy and content. I did and I was . . . for a short time. After college, I believed if I qualified for the Boston Marathon, I would be happy and content. I did and I was . . . for a short time. I then believed if I did the Ironman Triathlon, a grueling endurance event consisting of a 2.4-mile swim, 112-mile bike ride, and 26.2-mile run, I would finally be happy and content. I did (four times) and I was . . . for a short time. My point is that I was always striving for the next "hit" of happiness and achievement. When I took my focus off of the destination and learned to appreciate each step of the journey, I was able to feel as if I had "arrived" on a daily basis.

The happiest people, according to Ben-Shahar, are those who attach present and future benefit to their actions. In other words, people who enjoy a lifestyle that yields ongoing feelings of wellness will experience enduring happiness.

Transformation

We have been programmed to think about physical transformation in terms of how we want to look and what we have to do to achieve that ideal. Lasting transformation, however, is the result of how we think and, in turn, how we consistently act. Cultivating love and joy within is the key to transformation without.

When you set an intention, you create purposeful action by keeping your focus on the process of transformation as opposed to the outcome—consistency versus perfection. We often get fixated on transforming right away. We want it *yesterday*. However, in my experience, what we really want is to change the way we feel. The beauty is that changing the way you feel in the present speeds up the process by promoting more action! This simple shift in attention is the difference between experiencing happiness in the present moment and waiting for happiness to arrive in the future. Cultivating joy in the day-to-day process of transformation through positive thoughts and actions inspires you to feel good now. For example, if your intention is to transform your physique, consider taking your focus off of weight loss and discover the joy in walking with a friend or preparing and eating a nutritious lunch. Both are wonderful ways to move toward your intention while keeping your thoughts and actions focused on feeling good in the present moment. The key is to place your attention on the present benefit of your action. Why wait to feel good? Focusing on today's next positive action streamlines your energy by breaking your journey down into small, manageable steps while giving you permission to feel happy now.

Obsessing over outcomes can distract you from the process of reclaiming your power to think and act positively in the present moment. Cultivating specific intentions helps you create a harmonious way of living and achieving for a lifetime. When you make this shift, fear and self-doubt begin to recede and your whole power is awakened.

> " *Joy in the process is the magic, the master key to every door. Make the decision to arrive each and every day!*—Coach E

Success Story
Bruce

Bruce, one of my clients, experienced a remarkable transformation. When I first met Bruce, he described himself as a driven person who is used to meeting his goals. The challenge was he had a hard time adhering to a fitness and mindful eating program. He would begin, "fall off the wagon," and then try something else. Bruce was always looking for the next quick fix and never really found joy in the journey. He said, "I used to think that if I couldn't do it perfectly, I wouldn't do it at all. When it came to fitness and nutrition, it was all or nothing. Learning to focus on enjoying the process versus always driving myself towards an outcome has been liberating and transformative! The irony is the more I focus on enjoying the process, the more consistent and successful I am at reaching my goals!"

Your Turn

1. Take a few minutes to write down your fitness and wellness goals. For each goal, use the words "I intend to _____." _____

    _____

    _____

2. Write down the present and future benefits of your intentions. For example, if your intention is to stick to a consistent exercise routine, your present benefit might be the "feel-good" endorphins you get from a vigorous training session. Your future benefit might be feeling light and vital in your transformed physique.

    Intention 1: _____

    Present Benefit: _____

    Future Benefit: _____

    Intention 2: _____

    Present Benefit: _____

    Future Benefit: _____

    Intention 3: _____

    Present Benefit: _____

    Future Benefit: _____

This simple shift in thinking marks the beginning of your quest to transform. Your intentions will be the driving force behind your journey. Let's continue by exploring ways to cultivate the power of intention and how you can put intention to work for you.

Awakening Your Inner Genius

> *There is a life-force within your soul, seek that life.*
> *There is a gem in the mountain of your body, seek that mine.*
> —Rumi

The knowledge and power to break through does not lie somewhere "out there" but within you. Available beneath past fears, frustrations, failures, and limiting habits and beliefs is a vital life force that, when transferred into action, is unstoppable. I call this your "inner genius."

Genius, in this context, is not something gifted to select individuals or based on IQ. Genius is your innate ability to act toward your potential. This is a great gift given to each and every one of us. Remembering this gift connects you to an unlimited source of wisdom and power for your transformation journey.

Your inner genius can be described and experienced in many different ways, some of which include:

▶ an authentic inner voice or "gut" feeling

▶ an urge to take action

▶ an experience that causes you to feel joyous, unstoppable, or "in the zone"

Cultivating intention awakens your inner genius by aligning you with the source of your power.

Success Story
Jake

My client Jake discovered his inner genius by taking action. "My inner genius was sparked through reluctant action. My wife had been on me about exercising and losing weight. I was unmotivated and didn't think I had the time. When I began the program, I must admit it was tough staying consistent. However, I stuck with it and one day after a workout I noticed how energized and vital I felt. I was actually enjoying the workout! This was the tipping point for me. Since then I've often experienced my inner voice saying, 'Jake you *can* do it! You've done the workout before and you can do it again . . . stick with it!' I've come to rely on this inner knowledge to help me take consistent, inspired action on the days when I feel unmotivated. I now know the power to break through does not lie somewhere 'out there' but is within me."

Your Turn

Think of a time when you listened to your inner genius. Perhaps there was a moment when an answer spontaneously came to you or you felt compelled to take action. Describe that experience:

_____

_____

_____

_____

_____

Learning to consciously recognize and appreciate your inner genius will help you realize your true potential. The exercises in this workbook are designed to strengthen your personal connection to your inner genius.

Tune In to Your Inner Genius

> " *All you need is deep within you waiting to unfold and reveal itself. All you have to do is be still and take time to seek for what is within, and you will surely find It.* —Eileen Caddy

Actively tuning into your inner genius involves quieting your mind and focusing your attention on the present moment. The challenge is that your mind often draws you away from the present moment by anchoring you in the past or pulling you toward the future. What gets lost is the power of right now. The present moment holds the frequency of your inner genius. It's within the stillness of the present moment that your genius can be heard and felt. Often what keeps us away from claiming our power is the limiting mental chatter rooted in past negative experiences or future fears.

Negative mental chatter can immobilize you from taking positive action. Some classic examples include:

I can't do that.
I don't have time.
What if I fail?

Applied quiet time can move you through limiting mental chatter to the frequency of your inner genius. It can also give you access to profound states of inner peace, tranquility, and insight.

The Power of Applied Quiet Time

> *The intellect has little to do on the road to discovery. There comes a leap in consciousness, call it intuition or what you will, the solution comes to you and you don't know how or why. —Albert Einstein*

The intention of applied quiet time and personal contemplation in the context of transformation is to learn how to tame limiting mental chatter and tune into the presence of your genius. Quiet time is a powerful medium for awakening your power to break through.

The duration and skill of your practice will develop organically over time. Consistently taking a few minutes each day to relax and quiet negative chatter immediately puts you in a natural and powerful state of presence. It's often within this presence that your inner genius is experienced.

> *There is guidance for each of us and by lowly listening we shall hear the right word. —Ralph Waldo Emerson*

GETTING STARTED

Posture
Experiment with sitting (floor, chair, knees) or lying on your back. The intention is to use a posture that keeps your back straight, your body relaxed, and your airway open.

Attitude
Maintain an attitude of openness, non-judgment, and possibility. Regardless of what your past beliefs and experiences with contemplation and meditation are, give it a chance.

Mindfulness
Mindfulness means focusing attention on what you're doing in the present moment. In a breathing

meditation, you create mindfulness by focusing your full attention on your breath. Know that it's normal to have a parade of thoughts emerge when you begin to slow down. The way to detach from these "visitors" is to witness and acknowledge the thoughts and then return to your breath. For example, if you begin to think of all the things you have to do today, I suggest saying to yourself, "No problem," and return your attention to your breath.

Time

There is no right length of time for meditation. As little as two minutes of focused quiet time can be extremely effective.

Space

Designate a special intention space for your quiet time. This can be anywhere: a spot in your bedroom, a special chair, or even in front of an inspiring picture on your wall or desk that evokes peaceful and happy feelings.

BECOMING MINDFUL OF YOUR BREATH

1. Close your eyes and cover your ears with your hand. Take a few comfortable breaths and notice:
   - how deep, shallow, fast, or slow your breath is
   - the sensation of the air traveling into your nose
   - the rise and fall of your breath. Does the rise happen high in your chest? Stomach area? Lower abdomen?

2. Take a few deep breaths, filling your lungs and expanding your rib cage, upper chest, stomach area, and lower abdomen. Notice how this feels.

3. Move your breath from your upper chest to your stomach area. Notice how this feels.

4. Slow your breath down by inhaling on a slow 5-count, holding for a slow 3-count, and exhaling on a slow 5-count. Notice how this feels.

5. Now move your breath from your stomach area to your lower abdomen. One way to do this is to place your hands on your lower abdomen. This type of breathing is called "drop breath" and is often considered the most relaxing. Notice how this feels. Do you find that your upper chest and stomach area stay relatively still? Over time you may find that you intuitively gravitate toward this type of relaxed breathing.

MINDFUL BREATHING MEDITATION

Begin your meditation by breathing through your nose or mouth in a way and for a length of time that feels comfortable to you. I suggest you begin by focusing on one or more elements of the breath, such as:

- how the breath feels as it travels throughout your body
- the rise and fall of your lungs and lower abdomen
- the sensation of air passing through your nose and lips
- the pause or high point of the inhalation and low point of the exhalation where you are not actively breathing at all

If you experience limiting chatter, know that this is normal. I invite you to witness the chatter as opposed to identify with the chatter. For example, anxiety can lead to physical reactions within your body such as a headache, tight muscles, and shortness of breath. Often this happens not because of what's happening to you on the outside, but because of the way you internalize what you think is happening to you. Habitual negative thoughts can be experienced in your body and may contribute to disease over time. When you witness your negative thoughts, as opposed to identifying with them, they do not have as much power to weigh on your body and mind.

Like the rise and fall of your breath, negative and positive chatter comes and goes. Name the thought and let it go. For example, you could name it anxiety, fear, defeat, etc., followed by an inner reassurance ("No problem"), and then return your attention to your breath. Notice how this feels.

GUIDED RELAXATION

The following breathing technique is a simple way to relax, recharge, and heal.

1. Begin in a posture that feels right to you.
2. Spend a comfortable amount of time anchoring yourself to your breath.
3. Focus your attention on your feet. Notice how they feel. Are they tense? Relaxed? Tight? Don't seek to change how they feel. Just notice for now.
4. Begin to move up your body, scanning for points of tension and discomfort.
5. Once you've scanned your entire body, bring your mind's eye back to your feet. Slowly rescan your body, stopping at points of tension. Grant yourself permission to let go and disengage the muscles at the point of each tension. Notice how this feels. On every exhalation, allow your body to fall deeper and deeper into relaxation. Visualize yourself breathing positive healing energy into tense areas.

6. Spend a comfortable amount of time noticing, releasing, and breathing into points of tension. When you're ready, return your attention to your breath and spend a comfortable amount of time breathing into your entire body.

MANTRA MEDITATION

A mantra is a word or sound repeated to deepen concentration, support healing, and become present during meditation. Create a power mantra using one word for your inhalation and one word for your exhalation, or choose one word to focus on during both your inhalation and exhalation. Some examples include:

Inhale: *Love*
Exhale: *Anxiety*

Inhale: *Joy*
Exhale: *Fear*

Inhale: *Positive energy*
Exhale: *Negative energy*

OTHER APPLIED QUIET TIME SUGGESTIONS

1. Practice staying mindful in your day-to-day life. For example, when you do the dishes, focus all your attention on doing the dishes. If you find your mind wandering, return your attention back to your washing. Notice how it feels to be fully present in your everyday activities. Many people experience a heightened sense of focus and freedom when they practice mindfulness in daily life.

2. Use mantra breathing to bring focus and relaxation to a stressful situation. Concentrate on inhaling long, deep breaths on a slow 5-count and exhaling on a slow 5-count.

For a more in-depth guide to the art and power of meditation, I suggest five wonderful books: *Breath by Breath* by Larry Rosenberg; *Get into the Gap* by Dr. Wayne Dyer; *The Power of Now* and *A New Earth* by Eckhart Tolle; and *The Relaxation Response* by Dr. Herbert Benson.

REFLECTION

Take a few minutes to reflect on your initial experiences with applied quiet time.

_____

_____

_____

_____

_____

Questions: Direct Links to Your Inner Genius

" *Who we are and what we will become is determined by the questions that animate us, and by those we refuse to ask. Your questions are your quest. As you ask, so shall you be.* — Sam Keen

You are an unlimited and creative genius. You possess all the answers you need to transform. The key to unlocking the power of your genius lies in the questions you consistently ask yourself. Questions are the direct link to your inner genius in the present moment. I invite you to think of positive questions as personal guides that point you toward your intention.

For example, when you ask the question, *How can I find time to exercise regularly?* your inner genius immediately goes into creative overdrive, searching for empowering answers like:

- I can get up an hour earlier.
- I can take a walk at lunch.
- I can make a set time and date to meet a friend to exercise.

Conversely, when you ask the same question in a disempowering way, like, *Why can't I find time to exercise regularly?*, the voice of limiting beliefs comes up with all kinds of alibis and excuses about why you haven't made it happen:

- I don't have time.
- I'm unmotivated.
- I don't like to exercise.

The challenge for many of us is that we consistently ask ourselves disempowering questions that keep us disconnected from our creativity and whole power. Some common examples of disempowering questions include:

Why can't I get in shape?
Possible Disempowering Internal Answer: Because I overeat and I'm unmotivated.

Why can't I stay on track?
Possible Disempowering Internal Answer: Because I'm lazy and I never stick to anything.

Why is this so hard for me?
Possible Disempowering Internal Answer: Because I'm not as disciplined or athletic as other people.

Notice how each question is phrased. Typically, disempowering questions begin with a negative phrase like, *Why can't I ___?*

Simply creating a habit of asking yourself positive questions puts you in communication with your inner genius. Applied quite time can help you tame limiting chatter while asking positive affirming questions, and help you directly access and get answers from your genius. This is another simple and effective tool for accessing your power to make healthy changes in your life. The following is an exercise to teach you how to phrase your questions in a positive way.

Your Turn

1. Spend a comfortable amount of quiet time moving into a state of relaxation and awareness.
2. Make a list of some disempowering questions you ask yourself on a regular basis. Write down whatever comes up without judgment.

3. Next to each question, rephrase it in a positive, affirming way.
   Try using positive phrases such as:

   How can I _____?
   What's the next positive step toward _____?
   What would my future transformed self do _____?

Disempowering Question	Rephrased Empowering Question
1. _____ _____ _____ _____	1. _____ _____ _____ _____
2. _____ _____ _____ _____	2. _____ _____ _____ _____
3. _____ _____ _____ _____	3. _____ _____ _____ _____
4. _____ _____ _____ _____	4. _____ _____ _____ _____

The answers to your rephrased questions may not come up right away. Stay open. I'll invite you to circle back to these questions later on.

Anatomy of Intention: Readiness, Decision, and Purpose

" *At the center of your being you have the answer; you know who you are and you know what you want.* —Lao Tzu

Reaching what I call "a state of readiness" is a personal journey. When you're there, you know it. For some, it can take less than a second. For others, it can be a longer process. The key is to take purposeful action. Even if you're not fully ready, stay in the process. Stay active. With focus and consistency, like two sticks rubbing together, your inner fire will eventually spark.

When I began writing this workbook, my intention was to create a personal transformation guide that would inspire millions of people to take control of their mental and physical well-being. I genuinely wanted my vision to happen; yet, at first, I took very little action. I soon realized that making a commitment to the project was more than simply saying, "I want to create a revolutionary transformation workbook." I had to make a clear decision and commit myself to making it happen. Also, I had to allow myself to feel perfect and whole regardless of the outcome. Making the decision was uncomfortable. Frankly, I was terrified of failing. I had no idea how I was going to do it. Sitting with my discomfort, I asked myself *why* I wanted to write this book. The answer came to me quickly: I want to share what I've learned and make a positive impact on the lives of others. Suddenly, I had a clear sense of purpose and it inspired my next steps.

Knowing what you really want and deciding to fully commit with your whole self to your journey immediately puts you in a state of strength, expectancy, and resourcefulness. Making a decision does not mean you must have all the answers now; have faith that the answers will come. The moment you decide, things will begin to happen. Meaningful meetings, information, assistance, and inspiration will often appear in your life. These synchronicities are no accident. A clear decision connects you to the infinite knowledge and power of your inner genius.

The moment you utter the words "I decide," you reclaim your ability to take positive action. We often avoid making a clear decision because we fear failure and exposing our imperfections. However, imperfection is to be expected and celebrated! Your transformation program is a fluid journey. Being imperfect allows you to learn and grow. Setbacks and challenges can be stepping stones, filled with possibilities that can be used to make the next positive step on your journey. Trust that right now you don't need to know how. Have faith that the way will manifest itself. Be ready for all the resources that will appear in your life. Allow yourself to dwell in your whole power!

The first step is to decide what you want. If you don't know what you really want, I suggest you begin by focusing on how you want to feel. For example, "I want to feel peaceful, passionate, and joyful." Next, begin to focus on activities that will help you experience those feelings. Perhaps you are interested in starting a business, volunteering, or taking a class.

Once you know what you want, the next step is to turn your "want" into a clear decision. This is a signal to your inner genius that you intend to manifest your decision.

"I want to exercise regularly" can be rephrased as "I have decided to exercise regularly." This phrase change is subtle, yet extremely effective. Using words like *decide*, *commit*, and *must* help you take back your power and own your ability to transform.

After stating your decisions, you may not fully believe in your heart of hearts that you can make them happen. In addition, you may feel uncomfortable or scared. Allow yourself to have these feelings. We will explore the power of beliefs in Provision III. For now, the important thing is to make a clear decision, even if the "how" is not yet clear.

Your Turn

Whatever you can do, or dream you can, begin it. Boldness has genius, power, and magic in it. —Johann Wolfgang Goethe

1. Spend a comfortable amount of applied quiet time getting into a state of relaxation and presence.
2. When you are feeling comfortable and at ease, contemplate and write down everything you want to manifest in your life. Example "want" statement: *I want to complete a 5K running/walking event.*
3. Reword each "want" into a clear decision. Example decision: *I have decided to complete the Thanksgiving Day 5K Road Race.*
4. For each decision, think of two or more ways to keep your focus on what you can do to stay anchored to the present moment. Example focus statements: *I will focus on adding five minutes to my endurance run/walk each week. I will focus on how good it feels to exercise and give less energy to how fast I complete the race.*

Claim Your Power!

Now that you've made a decision, scream it from the rooftops! Tell the universe and awaken the power of your inner genius.

1. Read each decision statement out loud. Now read each one again a bit louder and with more enthusiasm.
2. Now say it as loud as you can five times with as much passion and conviction as you can muster.

How does this make you feel? Silly? Excited? Empowered? Scared? This exercise can evoke a gamut of emotions. Witness and acknowledge the feelings. You may hear your inner critic belittling your positive feelings. Ask the voices to kindly step aside and continue to focus on your exercise, repeating it as many times as you wish. Again, don't worry about *how* you're going to make this happen. Focus on what you've decided and committed to do.

Many people experience a surge of excitement and energy when they do this exercise. Bask in the possibilities. Feel your power!

The Magic of Autosuggestion

Autosuggestion is a simple method of conscious self-hypnosis that reinforces your intentions by reprogramming your subconscious mind to keep your thoughts and actions aligned with your decisions. This powerful method was developed in the early 1920s by French psychologist Emile Coue.

The Coue method involves consistently repeating your decisions in the context of an empowering statement while maintaining a relaxed and present state.

Autosuggestion starter sentence:

Every day in every way with the guidance, knowledge, and power of my inner genius I'm on my way toward _____.

Consistently instilling your decision into your subconscious using autosuggestion triggers the power of your inner genius. Remember, your job is not to know how this is going to happen. Your job is to get clear about the decision. Autosuggestion is a method of clearly telling your inner genius and the universe what you want and what you've decided to manifest. When you do, the universe becomes your supreme ally. Don't be surprised if chance meetings, "coincidences," or other empowering resources show up for you!

To create even more momentum, I invite you to take action toward your intention after using your autosuggestion. This action does not need to be big. The simple act of taking a bite out of a nutritious food item (such as an apple) or a single stretch or abdominal crunch will suffice. Anchoring your brain with autosuggestion and positive action can immediately put you in a powerful state of co-creation with your inner genius.

Success Story
Roz

One of my greatest mentors, my grandmother Roz, was a firm believer in the power of autosuggestion. She spent much of her adult life studying metaphysical healing and the mind-body connection long before it became popular. The book that changed the course of her life was *The Miracle of Metaphysical Healing* by Evelyn M. Monahan. I recommend this book as another resource on autosuggestion and other powerful techniques for healing and transformation.

Autosuggestion was the catalyst for helping her overcome binge eating and sustain her ideal weight for 30-plus years. The autosuggestion statement that worked for her was, "Today, with the guidance of my ultra mind [inner genius], I will effortlessly move toward my ideal weight." Using her autosuggestion kept her subconsciously focused on making choices that supported her intention.

Your Turn

I suggest you use your autosuggestion first thing in the morning and throughout the day when you need a boost.

1. Begin by combining your decision(s) with the autosuggestion starter sentence "Every day in every way with the guidance, knowledge, and power of my inner genius I'm on my way toward _____."

2. Next, spend a few minutes getting into a state of relaxation and presence.

3. Close your eyes and slowly recite your series of autosuggestions five times each. Some people find it helpful to tape-record their autosuggestions and listen to them while maintaining a state of relaxation and presence.

Select Your Power Team

" *Really great people make you feel that you, too, can become great.* —Mark Twain

Your power team consists of carefully selected allies who support your intention to transform. While you don't need a power team to break through, the right team can be an invaluable source of encouragement and inspiration. Ideally, the best allies are those who have "been there." These people know the mental roadblocks and have broken through them by learning to cultivate and unleash their whole power. Some allies may be on their own transformation path. Some may be professional coaches or healers. Others may simply be people who love and care about you. The goal is to create a community of people who will support you throughout your transformation journey. Here are some questions to help guide you in selecting your power team:

- Will they be compassionate allies?
- Do they hold your best interests at heart?
- Do they have a personal agenda tied to your success?
- Are they emotionally available?
- Do you trust them to support you without judgment?
- Do they have positive energy?
- Have they been there?
- Are they on their own transformation journey?
- Do they help create a supportive environment?
- Do you feel safe disclosing personal feelings to them?

Begin a list of prospective power team members. Keep in mind that your team may evolve over time.

POWER TEAM INVITATION

Become a part of a power team by joining my free fit and well online community. When you join the fit and well team you'll have access to my breakthrough exercise videos, nutrition tips, empowerment tools, fitness challenges, and more. Plus you'll have an opportunity to build camaraderie and community by interfacing with teammates from all over the world on our team website.

To join us go to www.coacherik.com.

SHARE YOUR DECISION STATEMENT

Share your decision statement or statements with each of your allies. I suggest you make an official time to do this. Make it important. Choose a private place and do it in person, or share it with our team online. Spend a few minutes getting into a quiet state of awareness. It's common to have fear. *What will they think?* Trust that your allies are not here to judge you.

While sharing your decision, stay connected to your feelings. When you're speaking from your head, it's easy to say, "I've decided to make better food choices." When you speak from your head, you lose your power. The key is to communicate with your heart. When you are fully present in the conversation, you may feel your body fill with energy, excitement, and possibility. This is your body acknowledging the awakening power of your inner genius. Sharing your decision:

- helps you gain internal leverage
- rallies support from your allies
- allows your authentic self to speak without shame
- makes your decision real

Personal Definitions: Success, Failure, Commitment

Personally defining what success, failure, and commitment mean to you frames your intention and awakens your power. *You* are in charge of how you think and how you react to your feelings. *You* get to make the "rules" of the game. *You* decide what it means to succeed or fail. This is powerful. Often, we give away our power by subconsciously plugging in to learned definitions of success and failure. When you base your success on your own definitions, you are in control.

Awakening your power frees you to experience success in the now. You get to set yourself up for feeling powerful, motivated, and successful every day.

Your Turn

Take a few minutes to think about your personal definitions for success, failure, and commitment. Write your definitions on the lines below.

Sample definition of success:

Success means listening to my inner genius and taking action. Success is about taking back the power to feel good about my body and feel good in my body. It means exploring my preconceived boundaries and accepting what I may at times perceive as physical imperfections. Success is about learning from challenges and setbacks. It means knowing that I deserve to feel confident and secure about who I am and what I have to offer the world. Success means celebrating my whole being in my quest to be a well-being. Success is a daily feeling of joy, knowing that I'm happily achieving and arriving while moving toward my potential.

Definition of success:

_____

_____

_____

Sample definition of failure:

I believe there is no such thing as failure. This is a no-fault program. External forces do not have permission to measure my success or take away my power. Setbacks and challenges are tools for learning, moving me closer to understanding what unlocks my potential. Knowing that I cannot fail is freedom. It motivates me to trust in the unknown and take emotional risks. No matter what happens, I can use challenges as positive fuel for learning and taking action toward my potential.

Definition of failure:

_____

_____

_____

Sample definition of commitment:

I fully commit to making my transformation program a top priority in my life. I've decided not to feel guilty if I'm not perfect because I'm already perfect and whole. I commit to learning and growing from challenges and setbacks and creating a space for my inner genius to be heard and felt without judgment. I commit to reclaiming my power to feel happy, confident, and successful every day. I also commit to moving toward the fit, vibrant, and empowered person I deserve to be!

Definition of commitment:

_____

_____

_____

Inspiring Purpose

> *If you cultivate a compelling enough why, the how will show up for you!—Coach E*

Ordinary people have done the extraordinary with an inspiring purpose: A mother can suddenly lift a car off her trapped child; a blind man can summit Mt. Everest; a woman who has struggled with her weight since childhood can lose 125 pounds and change the course of her life forever. The power to do the extraordinary is not something bestowed on select individuals. It lives and grows within each of us, including you! Cultivating the power of an inspiring purpose drives your transformation program by fueling creativity and igniting action.

I invite you to put the power of an inspiring purpose to work for you.

ASK FOR INSPIRATION

Inspiration is a moment that awakens the spirit of the whole you. To be inspired means to be in-spirit. When you are inspired, you become immersed in the unlimited possibility of the present moment. Some people describe an in-spirit moment as a sense of clarity, excitement, revelation, or motivation. Others describe it as a guiding light, a moment of awakening or innovation. Suddenly things make sense and become clear. An in-spirit moment fills you with the burning desire and courage to take action. It's a moment that allows you to see beyond your limiting beliefs and fears to the possibilities of your full potential. It's the awakened voice of your inner genius that says, "Yes I can!"

When you ask to be connected to the spirit, you attract inspiration into your life: a chance meeting, a kind word, a powerful experience. Asking puts the universe on notice. You begin to look at things a little closer and listen a little harder. Albert Einstein once said, "There are only two ways to live your life. One is as though nothing is a miracle. The other is as though everything is a miracle." When you believe and expect inspired moments to appear, you begin to look at life through a lens of possibility and optimism. That's the miracle. All it takes is one spark to ignite the spirit of your inner genius and awaken your power to take inspired action. Asking opens you to that intention.

As I neared the completion of the first draft of this book, I hit a period of writer's block. For the first time, I sat in front of my computer, hands on the keys, and nothing happened. After a few days, my inner cynic began to surface.

After almost a week of this, I decided to go for a drive and contemplate the future of the project. Without forethought, I remember saying out loud, "I can't do this alone! I need help! Whoever or whatever is out there, I ask for the inspiration to bring this project to fruition."

Almost on cue, lightness came over me. That night, I sat down in front of the computer. Without effort, my fingers began to type. I cannot tell you what happened that day to turn things around. I can tell you that the book you're holding now would not be in your hands if I hadn't asked for the inspiration and courage to find my voice again.

Your Turn

Take a few minutes to think about your intentions and the decisions you have committed to for this program. What do you need help with? What could you ask of your inner genius?

Here is an example of a request for inspiration:

I ask the power of my inner genius to connect me to the spirit. I ask for the courage and wisdom to find a purpose for physically and mentally transforming that is connected to my heart and inspires me to take positive action. I ask to be present to inspired moments that appear in my life. I ask to see life through a lens of possibility and optimism no matter where I am on my journey.

Write your request for inspiration:

_____

_____

_____

_____

_____

_____

_____

_____

_____

_____

You have now put your inner genius on notice that you're ready to be inspired. Keep on asking. The more you ask, the more you attract in-spirit moments into your life.

Remember to keep your mind and heart open to receiving inspiration. I suggest you carry a notepad and jot down moments that touch you. Listen to your inner voice. Notice how your body feels during different situations, experiences, and conversations. Feelings are a clear indication that your thoughts and actions are aligned with your inner genius. Often an in-spirit moment is felt within your body as a surge of feel-good energy or a shot of excitement. Some people describe this as an "aha!" experience. The spark can happen at any time, be ready!

NAME YOUR INSPIRING PURPOSE

Cultivating a purpose that fires you up means the difference between aligning yourself with something you *should* do and aligning yourself with something you *must* do. When you are mindful of your purpose for transforming, your mind and body move you to take positive action. Positive action in itself fuels inspiration—to act in line with your intention is to be in-spirit. Therefore, taking action creates the inspiration to take more action!

Your Turn

Spend a comfortable amount of time moving into a quiet state of relaxation and focused attention. Contemplate the following questions about your purpose for your transformation journey. Know that there are no wrong answers. Allow your inner genius to speak your truth as it is in the moment.

1. What is your purpose for transforming?

   _____

   _____

   _____

2. How do you feel when you think about your purpose for transforming?

   _____

   _____

   _____

3. What actions are you inspired to take when you think about your purpose?

   _____

   _____

   _____

Align Your Purpose to Your Core Values

> *To create what you want, you must act in line with who you really are.* — Coach E

The next step to cultivating a purpose that moves you to act is to align your purpose with your core values. Core values can be defined as those you prioritize and value most in your life. They act as a moral compass helping you make decisions and direct your actions. Examples of core values include:

Love

Freedom

Honesty

Responsibility

When you connect your purpose with your core values, you align your intention to the essence of your character. This inspires enormous action. The difference between action and inspired action is that action typically feels like work while inspired action feels effortless, exhilarating, and fun! That's because you're acting from a place of deep inspiration.

Your Turn

Spend a comfortable amount of time moving into a quiet state of relaxation and focused attention. When you are in a relaxed and focused space, think about your core values.

1. Write your top four core values.

    _____

    _____

    _____

    _____

2. Now write a definition of each of your top core values.

   Example:

   Honesty—to be sincere and speak the truth; to live a life that is free of deceit and aligned with the person I am committed to being.

   _____

   _____

   _____

   _____

3. Next, think about your decision, focus, and inspired purpose.

   Example:

   DECISION: *I have decided to transform my physique.*

   FOCUS: *I will focus on increasing my energy, not with a "quick-fix" fad diet but by cultivating a sustainable lifestyle that supports ongoing health, vitality, and wellness.*

   INSPIRED PURPOSE: *My inspired purpose is to emancipate myself from the guilt and shame associated with my body and past weight-loss efforts. I will allow myself to consistently reach for my full potential and find joy in the process.*

   Decision: _____

   _____

   _____

   _____

   _____

   Focus: _____

   _____

   _____

   _____

   _____

   Inspired Purpose: _____

   _____

   _____

   _____

   _____

4. How do your core values connect to your decision, focus, and inspired purpose?

Example:

Core Value	Connection
Love/Connectedness	My new lifestyle will give me more energy to be more active and have more fun with friends and family.
Freedom	Letting go of the guilt and shame associated with my body and past weight-loss efforts will give me the freedom to enjoy life and the process of transforming.
Honesty	Designing a lifestyle that supports my ongoing health, vitality, and wellness will give me the opportunity to live more honestly and aligned with the person I am committed to being.
Responsibility	Allowing myself to consistently reach for my full potential will help me take responsibility for my health and well-being. It will also help me follow through on other responsibilities in my life.

Core Value	Connection

Supercharge Your Purpose with Emotion

> *Success isn't a result of spontaneous combustion. You must set yourself on fire.* —Arnold H. Glasow

Think of a time in your life when you really went for it. What drove you to take action? What about that situation differed from others? What was the tipping point? Chances are the driving force was what I call "supercharged emotion."

A supercharged emotion empowers you to consistently take inspired action toward your intention. It's the emotional leverage that gets you out of bed on a cold, dark morning to exercise before work. It's the voice that encourages you to act when you feel unmotivated, unfocused, too busy, or too tired. It's a feeling of desire that creates an unstoppable momentum. It's your inner genius saying, "I'm ready to do whatever it takes to actively awaken my potential."

Your Turn

A thought aligned with intense emotion creates the internal leverage to move you into action. Using the questions below as a guide, supercharge your thoughts by dwelling on your purpose. The intention is to connect as much emotion to your thoughts as possible. Notice how dwelling on these questions makes you feel.

- What brings me the most joy in my life? How will acting in line with my purpose enhance that joy?
- How will happily achieving my purpose make me feel?
- What am I willing to do to happily achieve my purpose? How will my life be enhanced? Increased energy? Health? Well-being?
- Whom do I love and who loves me? How will happily achieving my purpose enhance those relationships?
- How will my life be different if I choose not to act in line with my purpose? How will it affect my energy, health, and well-being?
- How will not choosing to happily achieve my purpose affect my relationships?
- What are my gifts and skills? How can I use those gifts and skills to happily achieve my purpose?

- When in my life have I used my strengths and skills to achieve something important to me? What can I do to feel that kind of desire and passion now?

Seek the answers to these questions. A surge of emotion is a common sign that you're connecting to the power of your inner genius. Dwell on these powerful emotions and set your heart and intention on fire!

Whole Power Summary

In Provision I, you learned that intention is the genesis of action. When you set an intention, you begin to take purposeful action. Living with intention will connect you to the present and cultivate enduring happiness in your life.

Remember that you are a genius. The knowledge and power to break through is within you. Awakening your inner genius connects you to an unlimited source of wisdom and power for your transformation journey. Your inner genius can be experienced as an authentic inner voice or gut feeling; an urge to take inspired action; or an experience that makes you feel joyous, in the flow, exhilarated, or in the zone. The present moment holds the frequency of your inner genius. And focused quiet time can help you tune in to that frequency.

Knowing what you want and making decisions with your core self puts you in a state of strength, expectancy, and resourcefulness. Setting an inspiring purpose that is in line with your core values and charged with emotion will drive your program by fueling creativity and igniting action!

Provision II
Vivid Vision

> *What we plant in the soil of contemplation, we shall reap in the harvest of action.* —Meister Eckhart

A vivid vision is a clear mental picture that illustrates your intention to your inner genius. If part of your intention has to do with your physical self, a vivid vision may include a specific mental picture of the healthy, vibrant body you intend to manifest. If part of your intention is to feel more empowered and alive, your picture may include a vivid visualization of you making empowered choices and feeling explosive vitality. The magic is that your inner genius does not differentiate between what is real and what you suggest is real. Therefore, your vision acts as an internal beacon, magnetically pulling you (both consciously and subconsciously) toward your intention.

Body Image

> *The shell must break before the bird can fly.*
> —Lord Alfred Tennyson

Before setting your new empowering vision, it's important to be aware of your current body image. For many people body image is a loaded topic. As I said in the introduction, popular culture and quick-fix diet and exercise plans try to sell us on a physical "ideal" that is unrealistic for us. This often wreaks havoc on how we see and feel about our bodies.

The following exercises will help you understand how the image you have of your body contributes to your emotional state, physical activity, and overall lifestyle choices.

Once you realize the impact your body image has on your life, you can start to re-envision yourself in a way that aligns with the life you intend to live versus the life outside forces say you should aspire to live.

Your Turn

Close your eyes and envision yourself as you are in this moment. What do you see? Answer the following questions with as much detail as possible:

1. How do you feel as you look at your body with your mind's eye?

   _____

   _____

   _____

2. How do you physically feel within your body?

   _____

   _____

   _____

3. What do you like about your body?

   _____

   _____

   _____

4. What do you wish you could change about your body?

   _____

   _____

   _____

5. Take a few minutes to reflect on your answers to these questions. Did you find yourself going into negative self-talk mode? If so, what were you saying to yourself? Did you allow yourself to acknowledge positive feelings about your body? If so, what were you able to focus on that created a positive emotion or image?

   _____

   _____

   _____

   _____

   _____

For many people, this exercise brings acute awareness of how they currently feel about their physical selves. If you found yourself in negative self-talk mode, it's important to be aware of how this thinking can limit you from breaking through. Remember, your body image and vision are the mark your inner genius is aiming for. So when you say to yourself, "I am overweight," your inner genius responds in kind by attracting more factors into your life that contribute to being overweight. No matter how hard you try, a limiting body image will almost always prevent you from creating and manifesting a new vision by keeping you anchored to the old image.

Success Story
Lynn

My client Lynn's story provides an example of how transforming your mind can be the catalyst to transforming your body. Lynn had struggled with her weight since childhood. Using a popular diet, she lost fifty-six pounds and felt fantastic. The challenge was even though she had lost the weight, her mind held on to a body image and identity that supported being overweight: Even though her body had transformed, she was still programmed to think, feel, and act like an overweight person. As a result, being fit and vibrant made her feel more uncomfortable than being overweight. Over time, she subconsciously replayed old habits that kept her in line with her old body image and script.

By developing an intention that was aligned with her vivid vision of her transformed self, versus trying to measure up to an advertised ideal, Lynn transformed her thoughts and awakened her power to take consistent action. She lost the weight again and has maintained the weight loss for three years. More importantly, the image of who she is has dramatically changed.

Physical transformation does not always mean an immediate change in your body image. This is important to note, as many people are successful at creating change yet have a difficult time sustaining it. Remember, it's not just about what you have to do to sustain meaningful transformation, it's about who you have to be. You have to believe you deserve to be successful. Lynn's body image was stuck in the past even though she had lost fifty-six pounds. The breakthrough for Lynn began when she became aware of her limiting body image and how she supported that image with her habitual thoughts. As her awareness grew, she was able to break out of her shell by reinforcing that she deserved to be successful and creating a new vivid vision that matched her intention.

Clearly Describe Your Vision

> *Your vision will become clear only when you can look into your heart. Who looks outside, dreams. Who looks inside, awakens.*
> —Carl Jung

Describing a clear vision of your future transformed self can be challenging. You may have a hard time imagining your life as a fit, energetic, and empowered person, especially if you've never felt that way before. That's okay. Your vision will evolve as you begin to realize the possibilities of living your intended life.

Remember, every body is different and every body is beautiful! We're all genetically and physiologically different. You are a magnificent and perfect original. Remembering this truth turns your energy inward and helps you to create a vision based on a sense of personal connection, security, and individuality as opposed to some unattainable ideal.

The power of a vivid vision lies in the connection to how you feel. When your vision is in sync with your inner genius, you often feel a sense of clarity, excitement, and ease. It's all about you: what you believe, value, stand for, and intend to feel like. Your vision is not about "measuring up," but about getting to the core of who you truly are. This doesn't mean that you shouldn't intend to feel attractive. These feelings are normal and can be extremely compelling. The key is to take back your personal power by defining what attractive means to you.

As you move closer to your truth and power, it's common to experience fear, anxiety, and limiting chatter associated with letting go of your old identity. Stay courageous!

> *The person you thought you were is no match for who you truly are!*—Coach E

Your Turn

Spend a comfortable amount of applied time moving into a state of relaxation and presence. Review your statement of intention, decision, and inspiring purpose, as well as the core values and emotions that are aligned with your purpose. Using the following questions as a guide, describe your vision in as much detail as possible.

1. What does your transformed self look like?

    _____

    _____

2. How does it feel to be the transformed version of yourself?

    _____

    _____

3. What kind of activities does your transformed self enjoy?

    _____

    _____

4. What (positive) habits does your transformed self have?

    _____

    _____

5. What kind of relationship does your transformed self have with his/her body?

    _____

    _____

    _____

6. How does your transformed self handle challenges on his/her fitness and wellness journey?

    _____

    _____

    _____

As you cultivate your new vivid vision, surrender the natural desire to know how this will happen. Have faith and trust that the way will become clear. The focus right now needs to be simply on attaching a crystal-clear picture to your intention.

On the lines below, describe how your vivid vision is actually your true self uncovered. The way to know that your vision is aligned with your true self is by the way you feel. Does your description of your transformed self make you feel good, alive, and "in the flow"? Does it feel right to you?

_____

_____

> *One of the greatest joys occurs when you let go of who you think you should be and rejoice in who you are. —Coach E*

Create a Vivid Mental Picture

Now you are ready to create a vivid mental picture. Take a few minutes to reflect on your written description of your transformed self. Then close your eyes and cultivate a mental picture of your vision. Remember that it's normal to have negative thoughts as you do this exercise. If you find yourself going into negative self-talk mode, I invite you to be the witness, say "no problem," and continue on.

1. Notice if your picture appears close or far away. If your picture appears far away, begin to bring it toward you by slowly enlarging your mental picture of your entire transformed self. Notice specific details as you zoom in on your mental picture, such as colors, textures, smells, etc. Seek to use all your senses.

2. Staying focused on your mental picture, assign a specific movement or activity to your transformed body (for example, running, dancing, or playing catch).

3. Next, create a background for your mental picture. Focus on the details of your surroundings.

4. Bring your attention back to your body. Watch your transformed self move in your picture. Notice how your body looks when it moves. Notice how you feel. Enlarge your mental picture and bring it close. Slow your picture down, watching your body perform the activity in slow motion.

5. Keeping your attention on your picture, begin to notice how it feels to be your transformed self.

6. Now visualize your current self stepping into the picture with your transformed self.

7. Visualize your transformed self walking toward your current self in slow motion.

8. Visualize your transformed self and current self meeting and embracing. Enlarge your picture and bring it close. I invite you to ask your current self for permission to be replaced with your transformed self. Wish your current self well. Remember, it's normal to feel inner resistance. Notice what comes up without judgment.

9. Visualize the body of your current self slowly dissolving into the embrace and light of your transformed self.

10. How does it feel this time to see your transformed self in your mental picture?

11. Contemplate your vision and write whatever comes up without judgment. Remember, you deserve to be the intended version of you! It is okay if your new vision does not feel comfortable right away. Creating a new vision can be difficult and often happens over time. If it doesn't happen right away, no problem! You can always come back to this exercise later on.

_____

_____

> *When I dare to be powerful—to use my strength in the service of my vision, then it becomes less and less important whether I am afraid.*
> —Audre Lorde

Be Your Vision

The exciting news is that right now, consciously and subconsciously, your inner genius is in the process of creating "the way" to bring your vision into fulfillment. The next step is to expedite the process by consciously bringing your vision to life in the present moment. The key is to be your vision in the now. The great nineteenth-century philosopher and psychologist William James described this as acting as if you already are. Acting as if you already are creates the thoughts and feelings that are associated with your intended self.

Remember, your inner genius does not know the difference between what is real and what is unreal. Your genius responds to what you think and feel. When you think and feel like your transformed self, you are moved to take action and make choices in line with your vision. For example, if your intention involves losing weight, start acting like a fit person now. Be your vision until you are your vision. Choose to feel happy, healthy, and vibrant now.

Your Turn

Spend a comfortable amount of time moving into a state of relaxation and presence. Contemplate the following questions:

- If you were an actor playing the role of your transformed self in the present moment, how would you play him/her?
- How would you feel about your body right now?
- How would you stand? Walk? Talk?
- How would your body image change?
- How would you communicate with others?
- What new activities would you do?

Now think of five things you can do to support your vision.

Examples: I can eat mindfully. I can make exercise a priority.

_____

_____

_____

_____

_____

_____

Limiting Habits

> " _Habit is either the best of servants or the worst of masters._
> —Nathaniel Emmons

For most people, the greatest hurdle in their quest to "be their vision" is overcoming limiting habits. A limiting habit is a behavior acquired through frequent repetition that contradicts your intention and vision. For example, if your intention is to tone your midsection and you have a habit of overeating when you're feeling stressed, the habit could be considered limiting. The challenge is that breaking through this kind of limiting habit isn't always as easy as saying, "I'm not going to binge eat when I'm stressed." Have you ever told yourself that you weren't going to do something only to find yourself in the same old pattern a few days later?

Most people consistently revert back to old habits because, on a conscious or subconscious level, the habit serves them in some way. While it's usually obvious to see how the habit limits you, it can be a bit more challenging to uncover how a limiting habit serves you.

Success Story
Tanya

My client Tanya had a habit of eating a large bowl of ice cream three to four times a week after work. While eating ice cream isn't "bad," per se, the habit wasn't helping her move toward her vision. Her ice cream binges left her feeling guilty and out of control. To offset those feelings, she often deprived herself of food the next day. Tanya was stuck in a self-defeating pattern.

Tanya took the first step in breaking free of this pattern by honestly considering her motivation for binge eating. She realized that deep down she didn't feel as though she deserved to be successful—the ice cream was a way for her to disrupt her progress. Eating ice cream in the evening was also her reward for a hard day's work. It gave her comfort, soothed her feelings of loneliness, and provided a safe and familiar routine.

By using her whole power and the steps outlined below, Tanya was able to find ways to overcome her self-sabotaging behavior. She learned to nourish her body in a way that does not interfere with her transformation journey—and allowed her to enjoy the food she loves.

Break Through Your Limiting Habits

> *Emancipate yourself from mental slavery, none but ourselves can free our minds. —Bob Marley*

Step One: Get to the heart of the matter

The first step is to bring awareness, compassion, and healing to the emotions underlying the limiting habit. The courage to look within awakens your power to break through the limiting habit and replace it with an empowering one. After spending a few minutes getting into a state of relaxation and presence, I invite you to contemplate the following:

- What is your limiting habit?
- How has this habit helped/served you?
- What are you afraid to let go of? What will you have to deal with if you let go of this habit?
- Are you using this habit to keep you linked to your old identity?
- What are you giving up by keeping this habit in place?

Step Two: Channel your focus away from the habit you *don't* want to an action or habit you *do* want

Focusing on what you don't want attracts more of that into your life. The key is to focus your thoughts on what you *do* want. If you don't want to eat when you're feeling stressed, focus on what you do want to do when you're feeling stressed. Ask yourself, *What can I do right now to move me toward feeling more relaxed and peaceful?*

1. What new action can you put in place of your old limiting habit?

   _____

2. For each habit you intend to break, complete the following statement:
   Instead of _____ (limiting habit),
   I will _____ (new habit).

Step Three: Install internal buffers

Often, we are not completely aware of our habits. Have you ever been in a situation where it felt like you were on autopilot, acting in a way that contradicted your intention and vision? A classic example of this is emotional eating.

The key to regaining control is to create space between your emotions and your actions. An emotional buffer is a word or mantra, combined with mindful breathing, that gives you time to make an empowering choice. Some of my favorite emotional buffer words are:

Deserve

Control

Believe

Faith

Some helpful affirmations are:

This feeling will pass.

What's a better choice?

What would my transformed self do?

It will feel so good to stay true to my intention and vision.

I deserve to feel good and be successful!

When you find yourself going on autopilot, stop, count to ten, take three to five mindful breaths, and recite your buffer word or mantra five times. After you create the space, ask yourself the following questions:

- Do I really want to do this?
- Am I willing to make a choice, just for today that is aligned with my intention and vision?

Immediately implement your new habit. Notice how good it feels to be in control of your choices!

Step Four: Visualize and emotionally anchor your new desired action

Emotional anchoring is a technique created by Richard Bandler and linguist John Grinder in the 1970s as part of a transformational system called Neuro-Linguistic Programming (NLP). Anchors are formed when we consciously or subconsciously link a powerful emotional state to a specific sensory cue such as vision, touch, sound, or smell. Can you think of something in your life that triggers an intense emotional response within you? Perhaps a song, the smell of spring, or a photograph that reminds you of happy moments from the past?

Consciously anchoring a positive emotional state with your new desired action helps to displace the limiting habit and creates a new response that supports your intention and vision.

Anchor Exercise:

1. Spend a few minutes getting into a state of relaxation and presence.
2. Close your eyes and visualize yourself acting out a limiting habit.
    For example, feeling stressed and going to the refrigerator for a "food fix."
3. Now replay the habit in slow motion, only this time insert your new empowering response.
4. As you watch yourself replace the old habit with the new action, remind yourself how good it feels to be in control of your thoughts. Dwell on these good feelings.
5. Anchor feeling good to your new action/response by squeezing your right shoulder. Hold for five to ten seconds.
6. Every time you choose this new action/response, anchor it by again squeezing and holding your right shoulder for five to ten seconds.

I suggest you do this two or three times per day until your new action/response becomes a habit. It may take a few days or weeks, depending on how ingrained the limiting habit is. The more you anchor feeling good to your new response, the more automatic it becomes. Remember, old patterns can be persistent and deeply embedded. I encourage you to stay the course, no matter how long it takes. Have faith you will transform your limiting habit. *You* are more powerful than your habit!

For an in-depth look at the power of Neuro-Linguistic Programming, I suggest a wonderful book called *Sourcebook of Magic: A Comprehensive Guide to NLP Change Patterns* by L. Michael Hall and Barbara P. Belnap.

Whole Power Summary

A vivid vision is a clear mental picture that illustrates your intention. It serves as an internal beacon, magnetically pulling you toward your intention. A vivid vision is a direct call to action, awakening the wisdom of your inner genius to guide you toward your desired picture.

When your vision is in harmony with your true self, you feel a sense of clarity, excitement, and ease. Anchoring your vision to your senses brings your vision to life in the present moment and moves you to take inspired action. However, being your vision often requires breaking through limiting or self-sabotaging habits. The four steps to creating a new empowering habit are:

One: Bring awareness, compassion, and healing to emotions underlying the habit.

Two: Direct your focus away from the habit you don't want to the action/habit you do want. Take that action.

Three: Install emotional buffers.

Four: Visualize and anchor new action to positive feelings.

Provision III
Believe

> *Aerodynamically, the bumble bee shouldn't be able to fly, but the bumble bee doesn't know it so it goes on flying anyway.*
> *—Mary Kay Ash*

Henry Ford once said, "Whether you believe you can do a thing or not, you're right." This is often true when it comes to manifesting your intention and vision. Like a self-fulfilling prophecy, what you believe about your ability to break through and transform almost always becomes your reality.

Belief is the foundation of behavior. When you believe at your core that you can and deserve to be successful, you behave in ways that support being successful. On the other hand, self-limiting beliefs and fears create behaviors that keep you stuck in the past and prevent you from taking consistent, inspired action.

How Are Beliefs Formed?

Beliefs are formed by your perception of life experiences and subtle messages from family, peer groups, and media. In order to keep your beliefs intact, your mind searches for evidence to support them. Once your mind finds evidence that supports the belief or fear, it's often reinforced with positive or negative self-talk.

Success Story
Bob

When my client Bob began, he was struggling with his weight and wanted to transform how he looked and felt. The challenge was he had self-limiting beliefs that were blocking his intention to lead a healthy lifestyle. He believed that exercising was not enjoyable and took up too much time. He also believed that transforming physically meant depriving himself of foods he liked.

Bob's past experience with dieting supported his belief that he had to give up all the foods he liked in order to see results. The only time he felt successful was when he went on a crash diet, drastically reducing his caloric intake and completely abstaining from foods he enjoyed. But this kind of diet was a short-term fix that eventually gave way to old habits and weight gain.

We also uncovered that Bob's negative perception of himself was based on his experiences as a child. In elementary school, he was constantly teased about his body and always picked last for team sports. As a result, he often felt self-conscious and inadequate.

Bob reinforced these beliefs with negative self-talk. When thinking about transforming his body and lifestyle, his internal dialogue often began with statements such as *I'm fat* or *I'll never be fit*. Without realizing it, Bob had created a set of rules and perceptions that held him back on his transformation journey.

When Bob began to see that his beliefs were rooted in the past, he was liberated to take positive action to create new evidence in the present. With each small success, the old beliefs began to dissipate and his true, empowered self began to emerge. To date, Bob has completely transformed his physique, joined an adult basketball league, and regularly participates in road races and triathlons.

Beliefs reinforced with self-talk can create internal boundaries that regulate how successful we allow ourselves to become. For Bob, even thinking about transforming his body triggered a mental push and pull between his desire to change his lifestyle and his underlying beliefs about what changing would mean. When you take action in spite of history you allow the unlimited possibilities of right now to emerge.

Holding Pattern

> " *Though no one can go back and make a brand new start, anyone can start from now and make a brand new ending.* —Carl Bard

Self-limiting beliefs keep you in a frustrating holding pattern by creating a personal story that may not support your intention to transform. Like a limiting body image, self-limiting beliefs often direct your inner genius to take action that keeps you in line with those beliefs. In Bob's case for example, the belief that he could never be fit was supported by his perception of past evidence and reinforced by his internal dialogue. His beliefs made meaningful and sustainable transformation next to impossible.

Fear

> "Obstacles are like wild animals. They are cowards but they will bluff you if they can. If they see you are afraid of them, they are likely to spring upon you; but if you look them squarely in the eye they will slink out of sight. —Orison Swett Marden

Underlying most limiting beliefs is fear. Fear in this context is not the healthy biological fight or flight mechanism that protects you from mortal danger. Fear is the feeling of internal conflict and anxiety that holds you back from following through and taking action. The irony is that the object of fear is almost never real. While the fear feels real, the object of fear is typically created by things that happened in the past (past evidence) or what we fear will happen in the future (future beliefs). Fear is rarely based on the present moment. Therefore, what we fear cannot be "real" in the present. The catch is that we convince ourselves that the fear is real, or will be real, and we may become paralyzed or disconnected from our ability to act consistently. Some of the most common fears related to transformation include:

Fear of Failure

Fear of failure is usually based on the emotional pain of failing in the past or the perceived pain of failing in the future. Some common symptoms of a fear of failure include:

- Lack of Full Commitment: If you're afraid of failing, you often withhold full investment in the process of change. This gives you an emotional out because you can rationalize that you never really gave it one hundred percent anyway. This softens the emotional pain that might arise if you were to make a clear choice and then not fully "succeed." It becomes safer to not fully commit so that, no matter what, you never really "fail."
- Lack of Action: The emotional pain of not acting is less than the imagined pain of acting and then failing. This fear often arises from a self-image that is based on appearing and feeling successful at all times.
- Limiting Beliefs: The notion that past evidence predicts future results can also be an obstacle. Relying on past evidence to frame the future cuts you off from the unlimited possibility of the present moment. Remember, past evidence does not equal future results!

Fear of Success

You're probably saying, "I want to be successful! Why would I fear success?" For many people it's not success they fear, but the perceived burden of success. Here are some examples of perceived burdens of success:

- If I'm successful, what will I have to give up?
- What will success mean? I can't possibly sustain this level of focus or commitment my entire life!
- I've always been heavy. If I'm successful, I'll have to give up my identity as an out-of-shape person. Who will I be then?

When you're subconsciously fearful of succeeding, you often set up what I call "a success threshold." This threshold acts as an internal barometer, controlling the level of success or failure you're willing to allow yourself.

When you begin to exceed your threshold, a subconscious trigger goes off that creates discomfort, procrastination, and self-sabotage. This "success coup" is often fueled by not feeling deserving or worthy of success. On the flip side, if you move past your failure threshold, your subconscious trigger goes off sending the signal to get back on track by taking positive action toward your intention. You may recognize this push and pull between positive action and self-sabotage or inaction as the infamous yo-yo effect. Some common symptoms of a fear of success include:

- procrastination: I'll start tomorrow or Someday I'll _____.
- feeling guilty for taking time out for yourself
- periods of action followed by periods of inaction and self-sabotage
- fear of change: What will it mean if I'm successful? What will change? Will my friends and family resent me? What will be different in my life?

Fear of Having to Be "Perfect"

For some, making a clear commitment to their intention and vision means having to be "perfect" in their program at all times. This feeling can create a sense of burden and anxiety that can be overwhelming. Common symptoms of the fear of having to be perfect include:

- an all-or-nothing approach: If I can't do it perfectly, I won't do it at all.
- a desire to be in control but consistently feeling out of control
- a rigid relationship with food, followed by periods of binging
- the belief that you are not in control of your actions and must force yourself to be "good"
- a guilty feeling when you're "bad" and a controlled feeling when you're "good"

You Are Not Your Past Story!

> " *Nothing splendid has ever been achieved except by those who dared believe something inside of them was superior to circumstance.* —Bruce Barton

Relying on limiting beliefs and underlying fears to frame your current life prevents you from fully experiencing empowering evidence now. In other words, by bringing the past into the now, you get cut off from the infinite new possibilities of the present moment. Letting go of these beliefs and replacing them with new inspiring beliefs takes tremendous trust and courage. For many of us, letting go of our past story can be very uncomfortable. Who are you if you're not your old story? It's common to feel fear when you really sit with this question. What if you fully believe and fail? What if you succeed? Who will you have to be then? What will you have to let go of?

Regardless of past outcomes and future fears, each moment offers a fresh opportunity to support your ability to transform. Like a giant boulder rolling down a hill, there first must be an impetus for the rock to reach the tipping point. The same is true with the power of new beliefs. Reaching the tipping point requires courage and an active leap of faith. Making that leap can change your life forever.

Access and Challenge Self-Limiting Beliefs and Fears

Accessing and challenging self-limiting beliefs and fears is like standing up to a schoolyard bully. Even though you're scared of what might happen, you take action anyway. Remember, most self-limiting beliefs are fueled by fear, anchoring us to what is known and comfortable. Often it's fear of the unknown and our perception of what the unknown will mean that keeps us stuck. In order to break free, we must challenge our fear. As Mark Twain once said, "Courage is not the lack of fear, it is acting in spite of it." Taking action in spite of fear gives you the opportunity to create new, empowering evidence that supports your intention and vision. Regardless of your history or how many times you've "failed," the power to take inspired action lives within you. The precursor to action is the courage to act. This kind of courage requires giving yourself up to the unknown and taking steps in spite of fear.

Access Self-Limiting Beliefs

Simply becoming aware of your limiting beliefs and fears can awaken you to the truth that these beliefs and fears are unreal in the present moment. I invite you to unleash your personal power to act by contemplating the following question: What self-limiting beliefs do you currently have about your ability to transform? Next to each self-limiting belief, list self-talk statements of reinforcement that help to keep that belief intact.

Self-Limiting Belief	Self-Talk Statement of Reinforcment
1.	1.
2.	2.
3.	3.
4.	4.

Challenge Self-Limiting Beliefs and Fears

❝ *It's not who you are that holds you back, it's who you think you're not.* —*Denis Waitley*

Review your self-limiting beliefs and contemplate the following questions without judgment:

1. How have these beliefs served you?

    _____

    _____

2. What are the underlying fears associated with your self-limiting beliefs?

    _____

    _____

    _____

    _____

3. What will you miss out on if you continue to assume these beliefs are true?

    _____

    _____

    _____

    _____

4. How do your new definitions of success and failure challenge these beliefs?

    _____

    _____

    _____

    _____

5. Challenge each belief by completing the following sentence:
    I am confident that I can (behavior) *even if* (obstacle).

    _____

    _____

Keep in mind that you may not completely believe what you write right away, but be mindful of how this exercise makes you feel.

Positive Self-Talk

> The only way to make sense of change is to plunge into it, move with it, and join the dance. —Alan W. Watts

The way you talk to yourself reinforces your beliefs. Positive self-talk in the form of empowering *I am, I can, I will,* and *I deserve* statements counters self-limiting beliefs by connecting you to the creative power of your inner genius.

When you say and believe the words *I am* _____, your inner genius believes you are and bestows all you need to become just that. When you say and believe the words *I can* _____, your inner genius believes you can and bestows all you need to move toward your intention. The words *I will* acknowledge your power to take action, and this empowering statement puts you in control of your destiny. The words *I deserve* give your inner genius the green light to create boundless joy and success.

Self-Affirmations

Challenge self-limiting beliefs using the words *I can, I am, I will,* and *I deserve.* For each belief you previously listed, create an empowering statement, or affirmation, that supports your ability to break through and create new evidence.

_____

_____

_____

_____

Remember, if you're having a hard time believing your affirmations, that's okay. Stick with it. An affirmation plus new evidence forged through action will eventually redefine your beliefs.

Faith

> Take the first step in faith. You don't have to see the whole staircase, just take the first step. —Dr. Martin Luther King Jr.

You are not alone on your transformation journey. I invite you to let go of needing to know all the answers. Allow the infinite wisdom and power of your inner genius to support, sustain, and guide you. The universe meets those who have the courage to takes steps in spite of fear. Trust in the wisdom that in this moment your limiting beliefs and fears are unreal. Dwell in possibility. Stop thinking. Have faith and start acting!

Your Turn

In a relaxed state of awareness, think of a word or affirmations you can use to help you cultivate trust and faith in the present. Sample word: *Deserve.* Sample mantra: *I may not have all the answers now, but I have faith that the way will present itself.*

_____

_____

_____

Create New Evidence

> " *Knowing is not enough; we must apply. Willing is not enough; we must do.* —Johann Wolfgang Van Goethe

Creating new evidence is the key to breaking through self-limiting beliefs and fears. Often what we perceive as unmanageable or insurmountable paralyzes us. Standing at the bottom of a mountain and staring straight up can be daunting. However, having the courage to take the first step, and keeping your focus on the next small baby step, makes the impossible seem possible.

Access Empowering Beliefs

Spend a comfortable amount of time moving into a state of relaxation and presence. Contemplate the following questions without judgment. Listen for the voice or feeling of your inner genius and write down whatever comes up for you.

1. What positive/empowering beliefs do you have about your ability to bring your intention and vision to life?

_____

_____

_____

_____

2. What evidence do you have that supports your ability to create meaningful mental and physical transformation in your life?

_____

_____

_____

_____

3. What do you say to yourself on a regular basis that supports your evidence and keeps your empowering beliefs in place?

_____

_____

_____

_____

Focus on the Present

> " _Yesterday is history, tomorrow is a mystery, and today is a gift; that's why they call it the present._ —Eleanor Roosevelt

Your ability to break through self-limiting beliefs and fears exists when you are fully present to what is _now_. In other words, focusing on choices right now, in this moment, will support new, empowering beliefs and your ability to transform. We often relate to ourselves in the now according to what was (history) or what will be (future). Relating to the now according to the past or future keeps you stuck in old self-limiting beliefs, fears, identities, patterns, and habits that disconnect you from your whole power. What has happened or will happen has no power in the now. Intuitively we know this. The challenge is that the mind seeks to make meaning out of the fear of the unknown with evidence that has yet to happen. All of your power is in the present moment. This makes the now a place of limitless possibility. Each moment is a new beginning, an opportunity to surrender to what is, to have faith, and to take action. Keeping your attention focused on the present keeps you in your power and allows you to make choices from a position of strength instead of fear.

This moment is *your* life.

Your Turn

 You start to be it when you believe it! — Coach E

Spend a comfortable amount of time moving into a state of focused awareness. Contemplate the following without judgment:

1. What small step can you consistently take to create new evidence that challenges your self-limiting beliefs or fears?

   _____

   _____

   _____

   _____

2. What would you attempt if you knew you could not fail?

   _____

   _____

   _____

   _____

Success Story
Alice

When I first met Alice, she told me that she always dreamed of running the Boston Marathon. Every year she would go to the race, cheer for hours, and leave feeling inspired, thinking about how wonderful it would be to run the race herself. When I asked her why she had never run, she immediately launched into a list of self-limiting beliefs and past evidence that made her think that running the marathon was impossible. Alice's self-limiting beliefs included:

- I am overweight and my body isn't built for running. (We later uncovered that her mother always told her as a child that she was chunky and wasn't "built" for sports.)
- I've never run more than 30 feet and when I did, it hurt; I felt like my lungs were exploding! (past evidence)
- What if I come in last, or worse, don't finish? (fear of failure)
- What if I get into great shape, do the race, and then fall out of shape? What will people think? (fear of success)
- If I train all the time, I won't have time to spend with my friends and family. (predicting the future without evidence)

After cultivating her first two Whole Power Provisions, Intention and Vision, Alice was ready to challenge the self-limiting beliefs and fears that prevented her from taking consistent, inspired action. She came to me one day and said very clearly, "I have made the decision to make my dream of running the Boston Marathon a reality."

For Alice to break through, she had to stand up and face her limiting beliefs and fears. The first step was to access her beliefs. Facing her truth took tremendous courage and set the process in motion. The next step was deciding to challenge her beliefs and confront her fears. Taking a step back and cultivating her new definitions of failure and success put her in a state of empowerment and released her from feeling like she had to "perform."

While cultivating her Whole Power Provisions, Alice uncovered that the way she talked to herself had kept her stuck in an old, limiting self-script. Her negative beliefs and fears were fueled by:

- not fully feeling as if she deserved success
- negative statements
- a negative evaluation of her ability
- negative stories about her past
- negative visualizations when she thought of running in the marathon

Alice needed to feel deserving of success by creating a new, powerful mindset that reconnected her to the wisdom of her inner genius. Alice did this in part with positive self-talk, auto-suggestion, and the gathering of empowering evidence through positive action.

Once we identified what was holding her back, Alice had to have faith that the past evidence supporting her beliefs had no power in the now. Even though she couldn't fully see how she was going to do it, she had to trust that the way would be made clear and move toward her intention. She began by taking action and signing up for the race. This brought up a gamut of emotions, yet it set the boulder rolling. Alice was face-to-face with her limiting beliefs and subsequent fears. By taking small steps, she could confront her fears, realizing that they were unreal or blown out of proportion.

For Alice, the key was to feel successful immediately. The intention was to develop new, empowering evidence in the now with a program that was effective and felt very manageable. Alice found (as most of us do when we take focused steps) that she could do a lot more than she thought. On the first day, Alice ran to the end of the street. On day 6, Alice ran two laps around her block. By day 25, Alice was up to twelve laps around her block.

By taking a leap into the unknown, Alice began to challenge her old, limiting beliefs with new, empowering evidence:

She discovered her body was built for running and that marathon runners come in all different shapes and sizes.

She discovered she could run more than thirty feet without her lungs exploding. This created momentum, while increasing her self-esteem exponentially.

After six months of training, Alice broke through her self-limiting beliefs and successfully completed the 2003 Boston Marathon.

Whole Power Summary

Beliefs are the foundation of behavior. When you believe at your core you will be successful, you behave in a way that supports success. However, many of us carry around negative beliefs that hold us back. Underlying most limiting beliefs are fears. The most common fears associated with transformation are fear of failure, fear of success, and fear of having to be "perfect."

Focusing on limiting beliefs to determine your actions prevents you from experiencing the infinite possibilities of the present moment. Breaking through and creating new, empowering beliefs requires faith, courage, and positive action. Positive self-talk and autosuggestion counter limiting beliefs and put you in a state of empowerment and possibility. Creating new, positive evidence supports new, empowering beliefs.

Provision IV
Self-Care in Action

In order to create there must be a dynamic force, and what force is more potent than love?—Igor Stravinsky

Self-Care in Action (SCIA) is a decision you can make in the present to think and act in line with your intention and vision. For example, if your intention and vision involves physical transformation, SCIA may include:

- using exercise rather than food as a reward for a long day at work
- preparing a mindful dinner, sitting down, and lighting a candle instead of ordering take-out
- taking a walk instead of channel surfing

SCIA turns your focus inward by inviting the question, *How can I value and care for myself in this moment and stay aligned with my intention and vision?*

Sometimes self-care is confused with being selfish or ego-driven. This is often the case for people who identify with being a "caretaker" and take care of others before themselves. However, consistently loving yourself through self-care in the present moment opens you to the possibility of loving others more fully.

For many of us, self-love becomes conditional: *I will feel good when I look my best. Or, I don't deserve to carve out this time for myself. I have so many other responsibilities that come first.* I offer that self-love is unconditional and requires us to make choices that support self-care right now.

Most of us have become disconnected from unconditional self-love for various reasons. Often we seek to fill the void by doing things that do not reflect our intentions. While these actions can make us feel good momentarily, they never really fulfill us. That's because deep down these actions do not reflect what we really want—to feel happy, loved, and whole. Remember, you are perfectly imperfect! You are already whole, "good enough," and deserving of unconditional self-love right now, no matter where you are on your journey.

Acting from a place of self-love feels good. Feeling good is a sign that you're in-spirit and aligned with your whole power. This is different from a fleeting moment of instant gratification. Self-Care in Action feels good on a deeper level, catapulting you into a new state of possibility and power.

It's important to note that it's nearly impossible to make choices based on self-love all the time. In addition, sometimes you may make choices that feel like self-care, but are not in line with your intention and vision. I suggest making a decision not to feel guilt when you make these choices. Instead, create awareness and open yourself up to future possibilities by asking empowering questions such as:

- Does this action support my intention and vision?

- Is there a better choice right now?
- What would be a better choice in the future?
- How can I learn from this?
- What can I do right now to "right the ship"?

Your Turn

Spend some time relaxing into a state of awareness and contemplate the following question without judgment: What does Self-Care in Action mean to me?

_____

_____

Taking Personal Ownership of Your Happiness and Self-Worth

> *No one can make you feel inferior without your consent.*
> —*Eleanor Roosevelt*

No person or situation has the power to make you feel anything . . . unless you agree to it. As the famous Shakespeare quote goes, "There is nothing either good or bad, but thinking makes it so." I invite you to work on protecting your feelings of self-love from external forces, such as other people, situations, and the media, by reminding yourself that *you* are in charge of how you think and act. Instead of reacting to things that may have made you feel bad in the past, be the witness to things that are out of your control. To paraphrase Buddha, if someone gives you a present (in the form of a negative statement) and you do not accept it, to whom does the present belong? Keep in mind that nothing can make you feel anything without your permission. Staying aware of this truth empowers you to own your happiness and self-worth.

Tune In to the Frequency of Love

A wonderful way to get connected to the power of self-love is to actively send and receive love. The classic song "Magic Penny" rings true: "Love is something if you give it away, you end up having more." Giving and receiving what I call "love power" opens you up to the frequency of love and allows you to love yourself more fully. Contemplate the following questions:

- Whom do you love unconditionally?
- Who loves you unconditionally?
- What does it mean to love someone unconditionally?
- How does it feel to be loved unconditionally?

Take a moment to silently send your love to others. For example, you could send love to a friend, family member, neighbor, or to those who are struggling in other parts of the country or world.

Forgiveness

Another powerful way to tune in to the frequency of love is to forgive people who have wronged you in the past or make amends with those whom you have wronged. Forgiveness does not mean condoning another's actions; it means releasing thoughts of anger, resentment, and hurt related to the situation. Forgiveness can liberate you and others from prolonged suffering and identification with suffering.

Be complete with others. Finish unfinished business. This means making amends when necessary or telling people how their actions have made you feel. I suggest staying away from the "blame game." Blaming puts people on the defensive and diminishes the quality of the interaction.

Why should you carry around past hurts, uncomfortable interactions, and resentments that keep you anchored to the past? I invite you to "travel light." Why be a martyr and sacrifice your life for things you cannot change? Let them go. I encourage you to release yourself from the continued suffering of the past and open up to the unlimited possibilities of love in the present moment. It's important to note that it's normal to have a situation where you are not ready to fully forgive. If the situation calls for it, it is important to work toward standing in your whole power by forgiving yourself.

Your Turn

In a state of relaxation and presence contemplate the following:

1. Whom do I need to forgive?

_____

2. With whom do I need to make amends?

_____

_____

3. Am I holding on to anger? Guilt? What can I let go of?

_____

_____

4. How would it feel to "travel light" and release myself from all suffering related to the past?

_____

_____

5. What can I do to "travel light?"

_____

Feeling Good: The Love Barometer

Feelings serve as an internal barometer of how attuned we are to the frequency of love. My suggestion is simple: Do things that make you feel good! This is not limited to decisions around exercise and nutrition. SCIA includes all thoughts and actions that make you feel good in your life. The positive energy created by taking care of yourself and giving away love to others gives you the momentum to take consistent, inspired action toward your potential.

Your Turn to Feel Good

1. Spending time in places that _feel good_ is a powerful way to cultivate self-love in the present moment and connect you to your whole power. What kinds of places help you feel the most alive? List your top feel-good places below:

_____

_____

2. Doing what you enjoy also connects you to your intention and vision. What kinds of activities help you feel the most alive? List your top feel-good activities below:

_____

_____

Now, contemplate the following questions:

1. What needs to happen for me to feel good on a regular basis?

_____

_____

2. What are three small things I can do for myself today?

_____

_____

3. Am I in balance? What area of my life needs loving attention?

_____

_____

4. What's holding me back from Self-Care in Action? How can I "right the ship"?

_____

_____

I invite you to circle back to the Your Turn exercise on p. 13. Review your disempowering and rephrased questions. Does anything new come up as you contemplate these questions?

_____

_____

Whole Power Summary

Self-Care in Action is the impetus in the present moment to think and act in line with your inner genius. The key internal question is, *How can I honor and care for myself right now in a way that supports my intention and vision?* Self-love requires making choices that support unconditional acceptance, regardless of where you are on your transformation journey. Consistently moving toward loving yourself with your whole heart through self-care opens you to the possibility of loving others more fully and with more presence.

When we are disconnected from self-love, we often feel compelled to fill the void with things that numb us from uncomfortable feelings. While these actions can make us feel good momentarily, they never fulfill us. That's because intuitively we know our actions are not reflecting what we really desire.

Acting from a place of self-love feels good. Feelings of peace, contentment, and happiness are often signs that you are in-spirit and aligned with your whole power. This is your ultimate breakthrough equation!

Keep in mind that the subject of self-love is often complex and multi-layered. I suggest that you use this provision as a starting point for a deeper exploration of loving yourself unconditionally.

> *Keep your thoughts positive because your thoughts become your words. Keep your words positive because your words become your behaviors. Keep your behaviors positive because your behaviors become your habits. Keep your habits positive because your habits become your values. Keep your values positive because your values become your destiny. —Mahatma Gandhi*

It's nearly impossible to overstate the power of a positive attitude. It's not what happens but the attitude you bring to what happens that has the power to shape your reality and create your destiny.

A positive attitude is the decision to dwell in optimism and possibility. It's a liberating force that can free you from procrastination, doubt, and fear. Choosing to focus on the positive during the inevitable ups and downs of life keeps your mind open to the next step. Staying positive, regardless of what life brings your way, puts you in a state of resourcefulness and inspired action. Cultivating the ability to stay positive in the face of challenges is an invaluable tool for your transformation journey.

Habits of Positively Charged People

> *Our lives are not determined by what happens to us, but by how we react to what happens; not by what life brings us, but by the attitude we bring to life.*
> *A positive attitude causes a chain reaction of positive thoughts, events and outcomes. It is a catalyst, a spark that creates extraordinary results. —Anonymous*

Becoming a positively charged person begins with a choice to view yourself and the world through a lens of possibility. The following are habits of positively charged people and suggestions for infusing positive energy into your life.

Decide to Focus on the Positive

The great psychotherapist Viktor Frankl wrote, "Everything can be taken from a man but one thing; the last of human freedoms—to choose one's attitude in any given set of circumstances, to choose one's own way." Things don't often work out the way we want them to. Knowing this, you have a choice. You can either dwell on the negative and attract more negative into your life or dwell on the positive, immediately shifting your mind's focus to creating a state of resourcefulness and possibility. Positively charged people actively look for the positive in challenging situations.

POSITIVE THOUGHTS

Have you ever stopped and really listened to the way you talk to yourself when things don't appear to be clicking? As you've probably discovered while cultivating your beliefs with Provision III, how you think affects how you feel; how you feel often affects how you talk to yourself internally; how you talk to yourself affects how you act; and how you act directly impacts your ability to break through challenges on your journey. Negative thoughts and self-talk are like prison guards that hold your whole power captive. Positively charged people consistently think and speak to themselves in a positive and affirming way, especially when challenges appear. Deciding to stay positive no matter what keeps you aligned with your power and attracts the things you want into your life. Suggestions for keeping your thoughts positive:

- Keep your words positive. Notice how you're speaking to yourself and others. Are your words positive and affirming? Seek to make the adjustment and notice how your emotional state instantly shifts!

- Have an attitude of gratitude. Feeling grateful is perhaps the best way to cultivate a positive attitude. Being in a state of gratitude focuses your attention on the grace and abundance currently in your life. This, in turn, attracts even more grace, abundance, and positive energy to you. Try beginning each day with the question *What five things am I most grateful for today*? Allow yourself to really feel the abundance of grace in your life.

Surround Yourself With Positive Energy

Positive energy attracts positive energy. Positively charged people are sensitive to how things make them feel. As a result, they seek to surround themselves with people, environments, books, magazines, television shows, movies, music, and other things that make them feel good. Suggestions for surrounding yourself with positive energy:

- Take stock of the amount of positive energy flowing into your life. Notice how you feel when you contemplate this.

- What doesn't feel positive in your life? What or whom do you need to let go of so that more positive energy will flow into your life?

Decide to Be Optimistic

> " *The optimist sees the rose and not the thorns; the pessimist stares at the thorns oblivious to the rose.* —Kahlil Gibran

Optimism assumes that things will work out the way you intend and, if not, will work out the way they're supposed to. When you're optimistic, you assume and expect that you'll be successful. This attitude keeps you connected to your inner genius and open to possibility. On the flip side, a pessimistic attitude keeps your mind closed to possibility and your heart full of fear. Suggestions for being optimistic:

- When things don't work out the way you want them to, remind yourself that what you need is on the way.
- Renew your faith that you're exactly where you're supposed to be in this moment. Pessimism is protection from disappointment. Remember you can't fail! You can always learn and grow. Allow yourself to take failure and disappointment off the table.

Decide to See Setbacks as Opportunities

Your transformation adventure is a non-linear path with many twists and turns along the way. Some people see these blips as "problems," often getting discouraged and giving up. A positive attitude can provide a shift in perception. When you're positive, you no longer have to see problems as roadblocks. Problems simply become challenges that provide golden opportunities for growth and learning. Often the most successful people in any area of life are the ones who've failed the most. The difference is they see "failing" as an opportunity to see what's not working, thus moving them closer to discovering what does work. One of my favorite quotes to illustrate this point is from Thomas Edison: "Results? Why, man, I have gotten lots of results! If I find 10,000 ways something won't work, I haven't failed. I am not discouraged because every wrong attempt discarded is often a step forward." Adopting the belief that problems are opportunities releases you from the fear of failing. Granting yourself the freedom to "fail" without judgment or guilt is one of the most liberating gifts you can give yourself. There is magic in failure. Rejoice when the road gets hard. It's often in shining the light on our "problems" that the code to unlocking our potential is revealed. When challenges appear, ask yourself the following questions:

- What can I learn from this?
- What do I need to adjust here?
- How can I use this as leverage for moving toward my vision and intention?

Become a Wellness Revolutionary by Helping Others Feel Good

> *Practice random acts of kindness and senseless acts of beauty.*
> —Anne Herbert

I believe the greatest exercise you can ever do is to reach down and lift someone else up. Positively charged people seek to selflessly spread positive energy and inspire others. When you feel good, you want others to feel good. Even when you don't feel good, seeking to make someone else feel good can lighten your heart and lift your spirit. This doesn't have to be a grand act. A kind gesture, a word of encouragement, a sincere compliment, or a smile is usually all it takes to make someone else's day and reconnect you to your whole power.

Imagine this scenario: You're in a taxi and you decide to strike up a positive conversation. As a result, that taxi driver may now be in a positive space, which directly impacts his next customer. That customer may turn around and spread positive energy to the three friends she's meeting for lunch. Each of those friends may spread positive energy to three of their friends and it goes on and on. The point is that you can have an exponential impact on the world by simply helping others feel good.

I challenge you to join me in creating a wellness revolution . . . one person at a time. You can make an enormous difference! Suggestions for helping others feel good:

- Call a family member to tell her she's on your mind.
- Ask a friend to go for a walk.
- Bring someone flowers for no reason.
- Give someone authentic, hearty praise.
- Express gratitude to someone who has helped you.
- Reach out to a total stranger. For example, strike up a conversation with a check-out clerk or pay for the car behind you at a toll booth.

Your Turn

In a state of relaxed presence, contemplate the following questions:

1. How can you help someone feel good about themselves today?

   _____

   _____

   _____

2. How can you be of service to your friends, family, community, etc.?

   _____

   _____

   _____

3. What random acts of kindness can you perform today?

   _____

   _____

   _____

Whole Power Summary

This concludes Part I. As you've learned throughout this section, the power to break through does not lie "out there" but within you. By setting intentions, creating a vivid vision, believing in yourself and the possibilities, loving yourself unconditionally, and fostering a positive attitude, you will put your whole power to work for you.

I invite you to call upon your empowerment provisions during your 90-day transformation journey, and then carry your empowerment with you throughout your life. To do this you must exercise your provisions like a muscle. Remember to refer to your empowerment provision regularly as you proceed with this workbook. A daily practice or review of the ideas that resonated with you will help you integrate your provisions into your life and foster a deep, on-going connection between you and your whole power.

Your provisions can be applied at any time and in any area and stage of life you choose. Now it's time to turn your intention and vision into your reality.

I invite you to continue to cultivate your empowerment provisions by joining Coach Erik and the other fit and well tribe members online for free at www.coacherik.com.

Part II
Breakthrough Fitness System

> *Living fit is a mindset put into consistent action. It's a feeling of mental and physical harmony that spreads through your whole life.*
> *—Coach E*

Part I offered you empowerment tools for breaking through inner roadblocks and taking consistent, inspired action. In Part II, I will invite you to make your breakthrough fitness connection. The two go hand-in-hand and both are essential in your quest to live your most fit, vital, and empowered life.

The intention of the Breakthrough Fitness System is to help you create a personal exercise program that is fun, effective, and fits into the fabric of your life. To help you do this, I've developed a system that you can do at your health club as well as an express circuit that can be done in the comfort of your home. Both versions are super-effective and can be done separately or mixed and matched to fit your needs.

The Breakthrough Fitness System combines leading edge training techniques, such as interval training, dynamic weight training, plyometrics, anaerobic threshold training, functional training, Pilates, and yoga. The result is a supercharged program designed to give you maximal results in minimal time.

Some of the exciting benefits include:
* weight loss/weight management*
* decreased body fat*
* long, lean, supple muscles
* increased energy and vitality
* increased core and functional strength
* increased body awareness/body control
* increased cardiovascular strength and endurance
* release of tension and stress
* increased muscular strength and endurance
* increased confidence and self-esteem
* increased flexibility and balance

* For best results, combine your Breakthrough Fitness Program with your Vital Eating Plan in Part III.

How Does the System Work?

Your body naturally transforms when the need to adapt to new physical stimulus (exercise) is recognized over time. The name of the game is *muscle confusion*. When your body is confused, it adapts. The Breakthrough Fitness System is designed to help you create an ongoing state of adaptation within your body. You do this by consistently reworking the training variables of modality (type of exercise), intensity (how hard you exercise), duration (how long you exercise), and frequency (how often you exercise). All suggested training variables can and should be customized to your current fitness level. This will ensure your workouts feel manageable while your body receives the message to adapt and transform. Keep in mind this is *your* program. I invite you to make adjustments to fit your needs and time constraints. If you miss a day, let it go and pick up where you left off. Remember, this is not about perfection but about the creation of a fitness plan that you enjoy and can easily integrate into your life. The idea is to make a personal connection with your program.

For video demonstrations, guided home workouts, questions, and comments, I invite you to join the fit and well online community at www.coacherik.com.

Success Story
Silvia

As a busy professional and mother of two, Silvia let her fitness take a backseat in her life. As a result, she felt chronically tired, irritable, and uncomfortable. In her mind she had "no time to exercise." She was looking for a plan that gave her maximal results in minimal time.

The 90-day Jumpstart Program was a catalyst in helping her take time out for herself, and take control of her health and well-being. She now says she feels energized, powerful, and full of zest! What she discovered is taking time out for herself made her a better mom and partner, as well as more productive at work. She also realized that you don't need to spend hours in a gym to look and feel fantastic!

System Overview

The 90-day Jumpstart Program combines the five pillars of optimum fitness: strength, agility, balance, flexibility, and endurance. Each week consists of four suggested workouts, one bonus workout, and two rest days.

I've also created Fit 'n Fifteen Express Circuits for training at home, with limited time, or while traveling. This time-effective 15-minute circuit series can be done anywhere and requires no added equipment.

The key to any exercise program is consistency. Remember, you can customize the type, frequency, duration, and intensity of your workouts to fit your life in a way that feels manageable and fun!

Success Story
Peter

Peter began the Breakthrough Fitness System shortly after completing a rehabilitation program for alcoholism. He realized his treatment was missing a vital component: physical fitness. So he integrated exercise into his ongoing program of support group meetings, therapy, and 12-step work. He attributes his workouts to helping him remain focused on his total wellness—body, mind, and spirit. During the 90-day Jumpstart Program, Peter lost twenty pounds and lowered his cholesterol, blood pressure, and blood sugar levels. Peter said, "My self-esteem also improved. I slept well and looked better. I even experienced moments of elation and gratitude for the first time in a long time. For an alcoholic, these are no small gifts. My training is now a part of my lifestyle and a critical part of my recovery."

Training Intensity

Determining your optimum cardiovascular exercise intensity is a crucial part of getting the most out of each training session. Train too intensely and you may be left feeling tired and lethargic. Train with no intensity and you won't maximize your workout.

In order to find the cardiovascular intensity that's right for you, I suggest you use the Rating of Perceived Exertion scale (RPE).

Rating of Perceived Exertion Scale

The 10-point Rating of Perceived Exertion scale (RPE) was conceived of in the 1950s by exercise physiologist Gunner Borg. Dr. Borg designed this scale to establish effective training intensities, using an individual's perceived exertion as a guide. RPE is based on physical sensations such as breathing rate, sweat rate, and muscle fatigue, as well as a psycho-emotional estimation on how hard your body is working. While RPE is a subjective measurement, studies have found that there is a direct correlation between RPE and your exercise heart rate. Also, using RPE is a powerful way to enhance body awareness by focusing on the signs and signals of your body.

10-Point RPE Scale

RPE	Exertion	Examples
1	None	Not moving. Lying on the couch.
2	Extremely light	Standing up.
3	Light	Walking at a normal, comfortable pace.
4	Moderate	Slight pick-up of breathing rate. Could have a comfortable conversation.
5–6	Moderately hard	Steady effort yet very manageable. Could have a conversation, but it is less comfortable to do so.
7	Hard	Effort is increasingly challenging. Could not sing without change in breathing rate. Sweat rate may also increase.
8	Very hard	Could have a conversation, but it would be uncomfortable to do so for long. Increase in breathing and sweat rate.
9	Uncomfortable yet manageable	Requires focused concentration and motivation to maintain effort.
10	Exhaustion	Maximum effort that can be maintained for a minimal amount of time.

Reference: American College of Sports Medicine Guidelines of Exercise Testing 1991 (4th Ed.)

Set Your Baseline and Evaluate Progress

To help you consistently feel empowered, I invite you to use the wellness scale on the next page as a guidepost to assess what's working and what's not working yet. Keep in mind, focusing only on "the numbers" (weight, pounds lost, etc.) can direct your energy away from finding joy in the journey. The wellness scale is a 1 to 10 ranking of enthusiasm, connection to your fitness program, and overall feeling of well-being. Remember, numbers have no power to make you feel anything . . . unless you give them permission! The invitation is to exercise and evaluate progress without empowering numbers on a scale to make you feel "good" or "bad." I suggest you focus on how you're feeling and let your inner genius do the rest. Be assured that you won't need a scale to tell you when you're looking and feeling fantastic!

Number	Feeling
10	Serious about my program. Feeling energized and balanced! In consistent action mode. Feeling very connected. Thriving!
9	
8	
7	
6	
5	Curious, but not yet serious about my program. Feeling a sporadic connection. Want to make it happen but having a hard time taking consistent action.
4	
3	
2	
1	Uncomfortable, low energy, and uninspired. Surviving.

I invite you to check in with yourself each week using the wellness scale as a guide. If you find yourself at a 5 or below, circling back to your Power Provisions from Part I can give you a boost. I suggest spending time going over the provision that speaks to your current situation. Notice the shift in your energy.

Success Story
Joanne

Joanne was having a hard time reconnecting to a fitness program. Ten years ago, she was a college soccer and basketball player. "In college, I liked that all of our team workouts were planned for us. When that framework was gone, I had a hard time creating a plan for myself. What drew me to the Breakthrough Fitness System's 90-day Jumpstart Program was the daily plans, as well as the variety and challenge of the program. Having a plan was key for me. Once I got into the workouts, the customized intensity and diversity of exercises were catalysts for rekindling my inner athlete and taking my fitness to a whole new level—even beyond my fitness level from college!"

Sample 12-Week Jumpstart Program

	Monday	Tuesday	Wednesday	Thursday	Friday	Saturday	Sunday
Weeks 1–4	Upper Body Power Circuit and Cardio-Powervals	Cardio-Rhythm and Core Circuit	Lower Body Power Circuit and Aerobic Cardio	Rest or Active Recovery	Cardio-Powervals and Core Circuit	Bonus: Go with Your Flow!	Rest or Active Recovery
Weeks 5–8	Plyo-Pump and Cardio-Powervals	Cardio-Rhythm and Core Circuit	Fit Fusion Circuit	Rest or Active Recovery	Cardio-Ladder	Bonus: Go with Your Flow!	Rest or Active Recovery
Weeks 9–12	Cardio-Powervals and Core Circuit	Fit Fusion Circuit	Cardio-Rhythm and Core Circuit	Rest or Active Recovery	Cardio-Ladder	Bonus: Go with Your Flow!	Rest or Active Recovery

Weeks 1–4 Workouts at a Glance

Day	Warm-Up	Workout	Stretch
Monday	Mental Preparation Cardio (5–15 min.) Dynamic Stretch Power March Shoulder Circles Arm Circles Standing Trunk Twist Hip Circles Half Squat Leg Swing	**Upper Body Power Circuit** 2 x 10–15 reps. incline chest press 2 x 10–15 reps. power push-up 2 x 10–15 reps. triceps extension 2 x 10–15 reps. triceps dip 2 x 10–15 reps. lat pull-down machine superset 2 x 10–15 reps. pull-up or one-arm bench row 2 x 10–15 reps. side-front shoulder raise superset Cardio-Powervals Week 1: 8 x 45 sec. at a challenging pace (RPE 7–8), each followed by 1-min. recovery at a moderate pace (RPE 4–5) Week 2: 9 x 45 sec. at a challenging pace (RPE 7–8), each followed by 1-min. recovery at a moderate pace (RPE 4–5) Week 3: 10 x 45 sec. at a challenging pace (RPE 7–8), each followed by 1-min. recovery at a moderate pace (RPE 4–5) Week 4: 11 x 45 sec. at a challenging pace (RPE 7–8), each followed by 1-min. recovery at a moderate pace (RPE 4–5) Cool down 2–5 min. at a comfortable pace (RPE 3–4)	Yoga Stretch Standing Mountain Pose Standing Side Bend Downward Dog Cobra Modified Pigeon Pose Bridge Pose Happy Baby Pose Cleansing Breaths

Day	Mental Preparation	Workout	Yoga Stretch
Tuesday	Mental Preparation Cardio (5–15 min.) Dynamic Stretch Power March Shoulder Circles Arm Circles Standing Trunk Twist Hip Circles Half Squat Leg Swing	**Cardio-Rhythm** 3–5 min. build to a challenging to very challenging pace (RPE 8–8.5) Week 1: 10 min. at a challenging to very challenging pace (RPE 8–8.5) Week 2: 13 min. at a challenging to very challenging pace (RPE 8–8.5) Week 3: 15 min. at a challenging to uncomfortable yet manageable pace (RPE 8–9) Week 4: 18 min. at a very challenging to uncomfortable yet manageable pace (RPE 8–9) Cool down 2–5 min. at a comfortable pace (RPE 3–4) **Core Circuit** 2 x 10–25 abdominal crunches 2 x 30 sec.–2 min. boat pose 2 x 10–25 reps. Pilates reach to 10-25 scissor kicks 2 x 10–25 reps. abdominal bike ride with reach 2 x 30 sec.–3 min. core hold	**Yoga Stretch** Standing Mountain Pose Standing Side Bend Downward Dog Cobra Modified Pigeon Pose Bridge Pose Happy Baby Pose Cleansing Breaths
Wednesday	Mental Preparation Cardio (5–15 min.) Dynamic Stretch Power March Shoulder Circles Arm Circles Standing Trunk Twist Hip Circles Half Squat Leg Swing	**Lower Body Power Circuit** 2 x 10–15 step-ups 2 x 10–15 side step squats 2 x 10–15 fit ball squats 2 x 10–15 fit ball inner thigh squats 2 x 10–15 one-legged dead lifts 2 x 10–15 lying fit ball hamstring curls 2 x 10–15 one-legged pelvic lifts 2 x 10–15 reps. hamstring curl machine 2 x 30–90 sec. chair pose 2 x 10–15 standing calf raises **Aerobic Cardio** 20–30 min. at a challenging pace (RPE 7) 2–5 min. cool down at a comfortable pace (RPE 3–4)	**Yoga Stretch** Standing Mountain Pose Standing Side Bend Downward Dog Cobra Modified Pigeon Pose Bridge Pose Happy Baby Pose Cleansing Breaths
Thursday	Rest or Active Recovery Day		
Friday	Mental Preparation Cardio (5–15 min.) Dynamic Stretch Power March Shoulder Circles Arm Circles Standing Trunk Twist Hip Circles Half Squat Leg Swing	**Cardio-Powervals** Week 1: 3 x 3 min. at a challenging to very challenging pace (RPE 7–8.5), each followed by 2-min. recovery at a moderate pace (RPE 4–5) Week 2: 4 x 3 min. at a challenging to very challenging pace (RPE 7–8.5), each followed by 2-min. recovery at a moderate pace (RPE 4–5) Week 3: 5 x 3 min. at a challenging to very challenging pace (RPE 7–8.5), each followed by 2-min. recovery at a moderate pace (RPE 4–5) Week 4: 6 x 3 min. at a challenging to very challenging pace (RPE 7–8.5), each followed by 2-min. recovery at a moderate pace (RPE 4–5) 2–5 min. cool down at a comfortable pace (RPE 3–4) **Core Circuit** 2 x 10–25 reps. boat pose to scissor kicks (modified or full) 2 x 10–25 reps. jackknife/fit ball exchange 2 x 10–25 reps. seated trunk twist 2 x 10–25 reps. abdominal rope climb	**Yoga Stretch** Standing Mountain Pose Standing Side Bend Downward Dog Cobra Modified Pigeon Pose Bridge Pose Happy Baby Pose Cleansing Breaths

| Saturday | Go with Your Flow! |
| Sunday | Rest or Active Recovery Day |

Weeks 1–4 Workout Descriptions

WORKOUT 1, WEEKS 1–4: UPPER BODY POWER CIRCUIT AND CARDIO-POWERVALS

> *Forget past mistakes. Forget past failures. Forget everything except what you're going to do now and do it.*
> —William James "Will" Durant

Mental Preparation

Before you begin each workout, I suggest spending a few minutes getting centered. When little thought is given to getting centered, the mind often acts like a wild horse running in all directions, trying to pull you away from what you're doing. Taking a few minutes to get fully present will help you focus, maximizing your performance and the effectiveness of the exercise.

Spend a comfortable amount of time stepping into the present moment by taking 3–5 deep abdominal breaths and briefly contemplate the following questions:

- What do I intend to get out of this workout? How will I feel when I complete this training session?
- How will it feel to move my body?
- How will it feel to act in alignment with my intention?

If you don't feel inspired to exercise, I suggest contemplating the following thoughts:

- Exercise feels good. I deserve to feel good.
- This is my time.
- I don't have to do this. I get to do this. This is a gift for me.
- Exercise releases endorphins into my body, which will dramatically change my mood.
- Commit to this exercise session only. Tomorrow I get to make another choice again.

Contemplate your intention and notice the feeling that arises. Remember, you don't have to be perfect and this workout doesn't have to be perfect either!

Cardio Warm-Up (5–15 minutes)

A cardiovascular warm-up literally heats up your body. The key is to slowly increase your heart rate, using a cardiovascular activity that is right for you.

The benefits of a warm-up include:

- increased oxygen to your muscles
- increased ranges of motion and movement, which help to prevent injury
- increased circulation and blood flow
- increased mental alertness

1. Choose a cardiovascular activity that is comfortable for you. This may include marching in place, walking, jogging or running, biking, elliptical machines, or dancing.
2. Begin by moving at a comfortable pace (RPE 4) for 2–3 minutes.
3. I suggest including 2 or 3 x 40-second pick-ups. This means bringing your pace up to a moderate intensity (RPE 6) for 40 seconds, and then decreasing to a comfortable pace (RPE 4) for 20 seconds. Each pick-up should feel like a steady output of energy, yet still be comfortable.
4. Finish with a moderate pace (RPE 6) for 2–3 minutes.

Dynamic Stretch

Dynamic stretching is controlled movement that takes your joints through a full range of motion. This is the optimal way of stretching before your workout. Dynamic stretching helps prevent injury by increasing muscle relaxation, blood flow, internal body temperature, flexibility, and maximal range of joint motion.

Power March

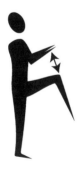

1. Stand and clasp your hands together with your elbows pointing out. Keep your clasped hands just below your collarbone for the entire set.
2. Drive your right knee up toward your clasped hands. The intention is to hit your hands with your knee. If you can't touch your knee to your hand, that's okay. Do what feels comfortable.
3. Repeat with your left knee.

4. Continue for 1–2 minutes.

Note: If you used this as your warm-up, proceed to the next dynamic stretch.

Shoulder Circles

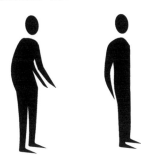

1. Keeping your arms by your side, bring both shoulders up toward your ears in a shrug position.

2. Slowly roll your shoulders back and around in a circular motion.

3. As you rotate your shoulders, squeeze the muscles in your upper back and neck to get an optimal stretch.

4. Make sure your rotations are slow and controlled. I suggest counting to 5 slowly for each rotation. If you finish before you get to 5, slow it down. Allow yourself 5 or more seconds to get the full benefit. Rotate your shoulders 10 times. Then, repeat in the opposite direction.

Arm Circles

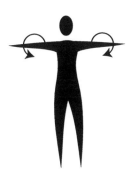

1. Stand with your arms outstretched.

2. Make large clockwise circles, keeping your elbows locked. Fully rotate your shoulder joints. Keep the movement slow and controlled.

3. Complete 10 clockwise circles. Then repeat in the opposite direction. Allow yourself 5 seconds per rotation to get the most benefit.

Standing Trunk Twist

1. Raise your arms parallel to the floor and keep your upper torso erect.

2. Gently rotate your upper torso by twisting from side to side at your hips. Do 10 rotations on each side.

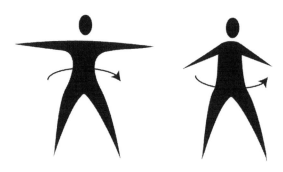

Note: If you have knee pain or a knee injury, I suggest you do this sitting on a chair or bench.

Hip Circles

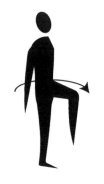

1. Stand next to a wall or chair with one shoulder facing the wall.
2. Place your hand on the wall or chair for balance.
3. Slowly bring your outside knee up to your waist as far as you can without strain.
4. Make a circular motion by opening your knee out to the side. Then place your foot back on the floor.
5. Do 10 rotations with both legs. Allow yourself a slow 5-count for each rotation to get the most benefit.

Half Squat

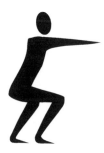

1. Stand with your feet shoulder-width apart. Hold your arms out straight in front of you.
2. Bend your knees and squat down 3–4 inches on a slow 3-count as if you are sitting in a chair.
3. Hold for a slow 3-count. Then, stand back up on a slow 3-count.
4. Repeat.

Notes: While doing this exercise, do not allow your knees to bend beyond your toes.

If you have a knee injury or knee pain, omit this stretch.

Leg Swing

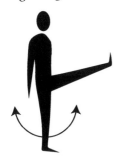

1. Stand next to a wall or chair with one shoulder facing the wall or chair.
2. Swing your outside leg out in front of you as far as you can without strain.
3. Allow your leg to fall toward the floor and swing it behind you as far as you can without strain.
4. Repeat 10 times with each leg.

Upper Body Power Circuit

The Upper Body Power Circuit is a streamlined workout designed to tone and strengthen your upper body, assist in the fat burning process, and release mega amounts of feel-good endorphins!

Circuit Suggestions:

- For each exercise, aim for 10–15 repetitions unless otherwise noted.
- Choose enough weight for each exercise so that you complete 10–15 reps with proper form.
- After each exercise, take 30–60 seconds recovery (or longer if needed) before beginning the next exercise.
- I suggest 1–3 sets of the entire circuit.
- Your intensity (RPE) may fluctuate during your circuit. While there's no suggested RPE for each exercise, you'll find your heart rate will elevate significantly during each set. The beauty is that you're not only toning and strengthening, but you're lighting your metabolic furnace for the next ten to twelve hours. So while you're at your desk or doing errands, you're burning calories at a heightened rate!
- The name of the game is intensity. To get the most benefit from this workout, you have to be willing to push it a bit. Listen to your body. Remember you can always take a break, catch your breath, and resume the set when you feel ready.

Incline Chest Press

Benefits: strengthens and tones chest and arms.

Equipment: free weights, bench

1. Select free weights that will allow you to complete 10–15 repetitions.
2. Lie on the bench at a 45-degree incline. Make sure your head and neck are firmly supported. Note: You can also use a fit ball or do a flat press while lying on the floor if you're at home.

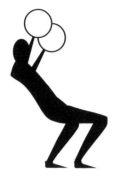

3. Firmly grab a free weight with each hand. Bring your hands up to eye level with your elbows pointed outward.

4. Tilt your thumbs slightly toward your chest. Your pinkie finger will be slightly in the air.

5. On a slow 2-count exhale and press your arms up, touching the free weights together at the top of the movement. Press your belly button toward your spine as you press up to support your lower back.

6. On a slow 3-count inhale and lower your hands back to the starting position.

7. **Repeat.**

Power Push-Up

Benefits: strengthens and tones chest, arms, shoulders, and core.

Equipment: floor, mat, or wall

Power push-ups are a fantastic way to keep your upper body and core muscles adapting and transforming. Choose a wall or floor for your push-ups. Begin with the classic push-up. When you can complete six full reps, begin to add variation to your sets. For each set, I suggest taking the power push-up to muscular failure, meaning the point at which you cannot perform another repetition with proper form. For fun, you may decide to keep track of how many reps you can do from workout to workout.

Classic Toe Push-Up

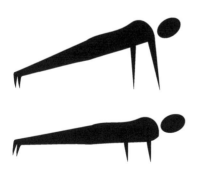

1. Lie on your stomach with your legs fully extended. Place your hands flat on the floor, shoulder-width apart.

2. Exhale and push your body off the floor. Keep your back straight and your head in line with your body. Use your toes as the pivot point, elbows fully extended and pointed directly behind you.

3. Hold this position for a 2-count.

4. Inhale and on a slow 3-count lower your body one inch from the floor, keeping your elbows close to your torso and pointed directly behind you. Do not allow your chest to touch the floor.

   Note: If you cannot perform at least six reps on your toes, I suggest you begin with the classic knee or wall push-up.

Classic Push-Up on Knees

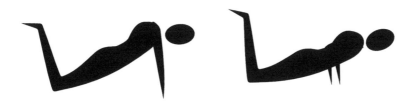

Follow the steps for the Classic Toe Push-Up, but instead of using your toes as the pivot point, you'll use your knees. Bend your knees at a 90-degree angle with your ankles crossed. Keep your shoulders and hips in line as you lower your entire body toward the floor.

Classic Push-Up on Wall

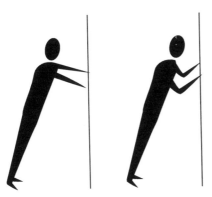

1. Follow the steps of the Classic Toe Push-Up, but in this variation you'll use a wall instead of the floor as your push-off surface.
2. Stand 2–3 feet from the wall, with your feet together. The farther away you are from the wall, the more challenging this exercise will be.
3. Turn your head to the side as you lower your body. This will help prevent injury to your nose if your hands slip.

Power Push-Up Variations:

Tight Power Push-Up

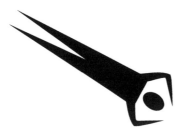

1. Place your hands on the floor 2–3 inches apart.
2. Keeping your elbows close to your rib cage, perform a full push-up, lowering on a slow 3-count and exploding up on a 2-count.

Wide Power Push-Up

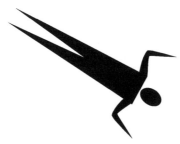

1. Widen your hand position 4–5 inches past your shoulder line.
2. Perform a full push-up, lowering on a slow 3-count and exploding up on a 2-count.

Decline Power Push-Up

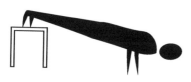

1. Place your feet on a bench, chair, or exercise ball, 2–3 feet off the floor.
2. Keeping your hands shoulder-width apart and your elbows close to your rib cage, perform a full push-up, lowering on a slow 3-count and exploding up on a 2-count.

Alligator Power Push-Up

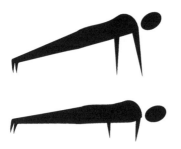

1. Begin with one hand just below your chest and the other hand extended 4–5 inches past your shoulder.
2. Perform a full push-up, lowering your body on a slow 3-count and exploding up on a 2-count.
3. Alternate hand positions.

Low Hold Power Push-Up

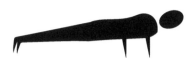

1. Begin with hands shoulder-width apart, elbows close to (or against) your rib cage.
2. Lower your body on a slow 3-count until your chest is 1–2 inches from the floor.
3. Hold this position for at least 60 seconds. Seek to increase duration from week to week.

Super Slow Power Push-Up

Perform a Classic Power Push-Up by slowly lowering your body on a five-count. Hold at the bottom (Low-Hold) for a slow 2- to 3-count and explode up on a 2-count.

Note: If you're not yet ready to explode up once you've lowered yourself to one or two inches from the floor, allow your body to gently fall to the floor after your 3-count low-hold. Then use your knees to return to the starting position.

Suggestion: Mix up the different types of power push-ups from week to week.

Triceps Extension

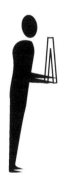

Benefits: strengthens and tones triceps.
Equipment: triceps pull-down machine with rope or bar attachment

1. Grip the rope (or bar) 3 inches from the bottom.
2. Roll your shoulders back and squeeze your shoulder blades together, opening your chest.
3. Lock your elbows against your rib cage and lean over slightly.
4. Exhale and slowly lower the rope toward your hips by moving your forearms and wrists only. Your upper arms stay completely still.
5. At the bottom of the movement, turn your wrists out and squeeze your triceps. Hold for a 1-count.
6. Inhale and slowly allow the rope to return to the starting position, continuing to keep your elbows tight to your rib cage and your upper arms still.
7. Repeat.

Triceps Dip

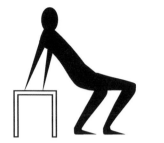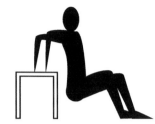

Benefits: strengthens and tones triceps, chest, shoulders, and upper back.

Equipment: chair or bench

1. Sitting on the chair or bench, place your hands next to your hips.

2. Keep your feet together with your knees at a 90-degree angle.

3. Lift yourself off of the chair, supporting your weight on your hands and keeping your elbows pointed behind you.

4. Inhale on a slow 3-count while lowering your body toward the floor until your elbows are at a 90-degree angle.

5. Exhale and gently push yourself up with your triceps on a slow 2-count back to the starting position.

6. Repeat.

Suggestions:

• If you find the dipping movement too challenging, I suggest you hold the up position for 10–30 seconds. Build up to 90 seconds in future workouts. Once you can hold the position for 90 seconds, begin integrating the dipping movement.

• To add resistance, straighten your legs or elevate them on another bench or chair.

Lat Pull-Down Superset

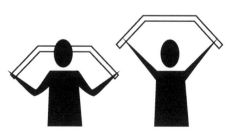

Benefits: strengthens and tones upper/middle back and biceps.

Equipment: lat pull-down machine with bar

1. Begin with your hands 3–4 inches wider than shoulder width. Lean back slightly.

2. Exhale and slowly bring the bar down to the top of your sternum by pulling with your upper back and squeezing your shoulder blades together. Hold for a slow 2-count.
3. Release and slowly bring the bar back to the starting position.
4. Repeat 10–15 times.
5. Then rest for 15–30 seconds.
6. Reverse grip, keeping your hands two inches apart.
7. Exhale and pull the bar to your sternum by squeezing your shoulder blades together, opening your chest. Hold for a slow 2-count.
8. Release and slowly bring the bar back to the starting position.
   Note: One set equals 10–15 repetitions of both grips.

Pull-Up

Benefits: strengthens and tones upper/middle back and biceps.
Equipment: pull-up bar or pull-up machine

Pull-ups are a tried and true way of building functional strength while toning and strengthening your entire upper body. Like the power push-up, vary your sets to keep your body guessing. See below for suggestions.

Note: If you're not ready for full pull-up sets yet, I suggest beginning with 1–3 sets of the arm hang exercise described in this section. Also, many gyms now have a weighted pull-up machine that can be an excellent way to do pull-ups with varying hand positions without having to lift your entire body weight. A fantastic alternative exercise is the bench row. (Description on page 83.)

Wide Grip Pull-Up

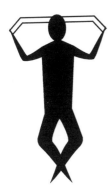

1. Begin with your hands 3–4 inches wider than shoulder width.
2. Exhale and slowly pull yourself up using your arms and back. Squeeze your shoulder blades as you ascend to ensure you're engaging your back muscles. Bring your sternum to the bar. Hold for a slow one-count.
3. Begin to descend on a slow 3-count until your arms are fully extended.
4. Repeat until you cannot perform another rep.

Close Grip Pull-Up

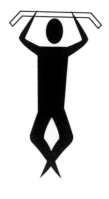

Same as the Wide Grip Pull-Up but with your hands only 5–6 inches apart.

Reverse Grip Pull-Up

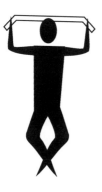

Same as the Wide Grip Pull-Up but with your hands reversed, pinkies 1–2 inches apart.

Arm Hang

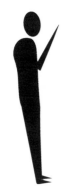

1. Place your hands on the bar, shoulder-width apart. If the bar is too high, I suggest using a chair or bench.
2. Begin with your sternum touching the bar.
3. Hold for as long as you can.
4. When you can comfortably hold your position for 60 seconds, begin to integrate one set of wide grip pull-ups into your workout—as many as you can do.

One-Arm Bench Row

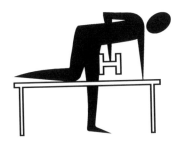

Equipment: bench, free weight

1. Place your right hand and right knee on a flat bench, keeping your back flat and parallel to the floor.
2. With your left arm, raise your free weight on a slow 2-count just below your armpit, keeping your left arm tight to your ribcage and your elbow pointed directly behind you.
3. Hold for a slow 3-count and then lower on a slow 2-count.
4. Repeat for 10–15 repetitions on each side.

Side-Front Shoulder Raise Superset

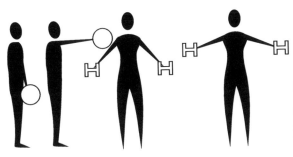

Benefits: strengthens and tones shoulders and upper back.

Equipment: bench, free weight

1. Begin by standing with your feet shoulder-width apart with a free weight in each hand.
2. With your arms relaxed by your side, create a 90-degree angle at your elbows with your knuckles pointed forward.
3. Exhale and begin to raise your elbows toward your earlobes on a slow 3-count. Squeeze your shoulder blades together. When your elbows are in-line with your earlobes, hold for a slow 2-count. Inhale as you lower your elbows toward your hips on a slow 3-count.
4. Bring the weights toward your nose on a slow 2-count. Keep the head of the weights pointed toward the sky. Hold for a 3-count and bring your elbows back to your side on a slow 3-count.
5. Repeat.

After you complete the last set of your circuit, I suggest taking 2–5 minutes of recovery and then proceeding to your Cardio-Powervals set. An optimal time to do your Powervals is after your circuit, especially if your intention is to burn body fat. The reason for this is that your body becomes depleted of glycogen (food that has been broken down into sugar and used as a primary energy source) during your circuit. As a result, your body becomes primed to utilize triglycerides (body fat) as a primary fuel source during your Powervals. In other words, you burn more fat by doing your cardio after your circuit.

Frequently Asked Questions

Q: Will the Power Circuits make me big and bulky?

A: No. In addition to maximizing caloric burn, increasing your Basal Metabolic Rate (the number of calories you burn 10–12 hours after you exercise) and increasing your strength, the Power Circuit is designed to increase lean muscle mass and tone.

Q: What if I have limitations and can't do a particular movement?

A: If the movement or modified movement does not feel right to you, I suggest omitting it from your program. Remember, the key is to discover the exercises and workouts that resonate with you. The same holds true if you want to add exercises to your workout. Mixing things up is a fantastic way to keep your body in a state of confusion and adaptation!

Cardio-Powervals

Cardio-Powervals are based on the science of interval training. Interval training consists of variable segments of high- and low-intensity cardiovascular exercise. An example of a short cardiovascular interval is walking at a relaxed pace for three minutes and then increasing to a fast-paced walk for one minute, and then returning to a relaxed-paced walk for three minutes. In this case, the fast-paced walk would be considered the interval segment. The Cardio-Powervals component of this workout consists of a series of interval segments ranging from thirty seconds to one minute.

A recent study by Jason Talanian, Ph.D., published in the *Journal of Applied Physiology*, suggests that intervals can:

- improve your ability to burn body fat
- increase your endurance
- increase your muscle resistance to fatigue

1. Choose a cardiovascular activity that *feels* right for you. This can be anything that elevates your heart rate. Remember the suggested RPE range for your intervals are *your* interpretation of exercise intensity. (Review RPE Chart.)
2. Adjust the duration and intensity of your intervals to fit your needs and fitness level. I suggest you start conservatively. As always, customize your workout to fit your needs that day.

Week 1

1. Choose a cardio activity such as running, jogging, or elliptical. Then complete 8 x 45-second Powervals at a challenging pace (RPE 7–8). Follow each Powerval with a one-minute recovery at a moderate pace (RPE 4–5).
2. After completing all eight Powervals, cool down for 2–5 minutes at a comfortable pace (RPE 3–4).

Week 2

1. Choose a cardio activity. Then complete 9 x 45-second Powervals at a challenging pace (RPE 7–8). Follow each Powerval with a 30-second recovery at a moderate pace (RPE 4–5).
2. Cool down for 2–5 minutes at a comfortable pace (RPE 3–4).

Week 3

1. Choose a cardio activity. Then complete 10 x 45-second Powervals at a challenging pace (RPE 7–8). Follow each Powerval with a 30-second recovery at a moderate pace (RPE 4–5).
2. Cool down for 2–5 minutes at a comfortable pace (RPE 3–4).

Week 4

1. Choose a cardio activity. Then complete 11 x 45-second Powervals at a challenging pace (RPE 7–8). Follow each Powerval with a 30-second recovery at a moderate pace (RPE 4–5).
2. Cool down for 2–5 minutes at a comfortable pace (RPE 3-4).

Frequently Asked Question

Q: Some of the Cardio-Powerval sets seem a bit intense for me. How do you suggest I customize the workouts?

A: Choose a moderate yet challenging intensity and then hold that pace for the amount of time that feels right to you. When you feel ready, begin to include Powervals into your workout.

Yoga Stretch

Equipment: towel, mat

After you complete your Powervals, try bringing your session to a close with a gentle yoga stretch. Yoga is an ancient Hindu philosophy and method to become one with your natural state. The word *yoga* means union with the divine or highest self. For thousands of years, yoga has been practiced for health, wellness, and self-understanding.

There are many disciplines of yoga that emphasize different practices to develop health of body, mind, and spirit through holding certain body postures called *asanas*.

A comprehensive exploration of yoga philosophy and practice, including advanced poses and meditations, is beyond the scope of this workbook. However, the following yoga stretches are a wonderful way to begin a practice, develop concentration, and bring balance to the other workouts in your program. To integrate a more in-depth yoga study into your program, I recommend taking classes at your local yoga studio or gym. You may also like to purchase a yoga DVD and practice at home; the Rodney Yee DVD series distributed by Gaiam (www.gaiam.com) is an excellent place to start.

Note: A more extensive yoga stretch is described on pages 104–115 as an option for Active Recovery or Bonus Go with Your Flow! workouts.

Standing Mountain Pose

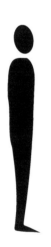

Benefits: balance, posture, alignment, and stretches entire back.

1. Stand with your feet together and your hands by your side.
2. Raise your toes off the floor, fan them out, and then gently place them back on the floor.
3. Feel how your heels, the outside of your feet, and the balls of your feet connect with the floor.
4. Tilt your pelvic bone forward.
5. Lift your chest up and out. Roll your shoulders back.
6. Raise the crown of your head toward the ceiling.
7. Inhale and reach your arms to the sky, keeping space between your fingers. Elongate your spine and arms. Feel your body lengthening.
8. Hold this pose for 5 or more breaths.

Standing Side Bend

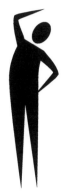

Benefits: increases flexibility in the spine, arms, and rib cage; aligns spinal column; opens lungs to increase oxygen intake.

1. From Standing Mountain Pose, place your right hand on your hip.
2. Raise your left arm straight up, creating a line from your foot to fingertips.
3. Bend your upper body to the right without forcing the bend. Feel your back and arm muscles stretching.
4. Hold this pose for 5 or more breaths.
5. Repeat on the other side.

Downward Dog

Benefits: stretches and strengthens your whole body and helps relieve lower back pain.

1. Begin on your hands and knees with your wrists under your shoulders and your knees under your hips.
2. Exhale and lift your tail up by straightening your legs and keeping a slight bend at your knees.
3. Press your heels toward the floor. Distribute your weight to your legs by pushing off with your fingers and palms.
4. Let your head hang naturally. Spread your shoulder blades away from your ears, opening up your collarbone.
5. Hold for 5 or more breaths.

Cobra

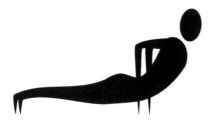

Benefits: stretches back muscles, abdomen, and upper body.

1. Begin by lying on your stomach.
2. Place your hands on the floor, parallel to your pectoral muscles.
3. Keep your toes pointed, with the tops of your toes on the floor.
4. Inhale and slide your chest forward, keeping your hands in the same position.
5. Roll your shoulders back and lift your chest higher, keeping your lower ribs on the floor and your neck in a neutral position.
6. Hold for 5 or more breaths.

Suggestion: Straighten your arms and gently lift your pelvis and quadriceps off the floor into Upward Facing Dog for a more advanced stretch.

Bridge Pose

Benefits: stretches and strengthens lower back.

1. Lie on your back and bend your knees with your feet on the floor.
2. Press your feet into the floor, driving your pelvis toward the sky.
3. Clasp your hands under your buttocks and pull them down toward your feet.
4. Lift your chin and press the top of your sternum toward your chin.
5. Hold for 5 or more breaths.

Modified Pigeon Pose

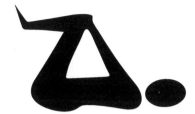

Benefits: Stretches gluteus, hip joint, and muscles connecting to the lower back.

1. Lie down on your back and bend your knees with your feet on the floor.
2. Cross your right leg over your left so your right ankle rests just below your left knee.
3. Hold your left thigh with both hands and gently pull your leg toward you until you feel a stretch in your right gluteus and outer thigh.
4. Hold for 5 or more breaths.
5. Repeat with your other leg.

Happy Baby Pose

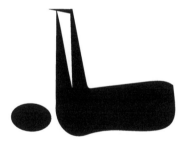

Benefits: stretches lower back and upper thighs.

1. Lie on your back.
2. Bring your legs up to your hips, knees bent.
3. Clasp your hands on the tops of your shins or feet and bring your knees toward your shoulders.
4. Pull your knees closer, feeling the stretch in your lower back.
5. Hold for 5 or more breaths.

Cleansing Breaths

Benefits: a relaxing way to bring your workout to a close.

1. Begin in Mountain Pose.
2. Exhale and swan dive down toward the floor, bending at your waist. Allow your knees to bend so that you're not putting pressure on your lower back.
3. Inhale and sweep your arms back up as you return to Mountain Pose.
4. Repeat for 5 or more breaths.

WORKOUT 2, WEEKS 1–4: CARDIO-RHYTHM AND CORE CIRCUIT

Wherever you go, go with all your heart.
—*Confucius*

Cardio-Rhythm is based on the science of anaerobic threshold training (AT). Your anaerobic threshold can be defined simply as a comfortably hard to very hard cardiovascular effort where your ability to have an easy conversation becomes increasingly challenging.

Exercising around your anaerobic threshold has tremendous benefits:

- maximizes fat burning
- decreases blood pressure and cholesterol
- helps manage blood sugar
- boosts cardiovascular strength and endurance

Choose a cardiovascular activity that feels right to you. The intention of this workout is to maintain a challenging yet manageable effort for an increasingly long period of time. While suggestions are given, the intensity and duration of each workout is up to you. Customize it and make it your own. Also, it's important to remember that your pace during this workout will likely differ from the Cardio-Powervals workout. For example, a challenging pace of RPE 8 during a 45-second Powerval will probably be a higher intensity than a challenging pace of RPE 8 during a 15-minute Cardio-Rhythm threshold segment. In addition, your intensity may fluctuate during a given segment.

Warm-Up (See Mental Preparation, Cardio Warm-Up, and Dynamic Stretch, pages 71–75.)

Cardio-Rhythm

Week 1

1. Choose a cardio activity. Take 3–5 minutes to slowly build up to a challenging to a very challenging pace (RPE 8–8.5).
2. Continue for 10 minutes at a challenging to a very challenging pace (RPE 8–8.5).
3. Cool down for 2–5 minutes at a comfortable pace (RPE 3–4).

Week 2

1. Choose a cardio activity. Take 3–5 minutes to slowly build up to a challenging to a very challenging pace (RPE 8–8.5).
2. Continue for 13 minutes at a challenging to a very challenging pace (RPE 8–8.5).
3. Cool down for 2–5 minutes at a comfortable pace (RPE 3–4).

Week 3

1. Choose a cardio activity. Take 3–5 minutes to slowly build up to a challenging to an uncomfortable yet manageable pace (RPE 8–9).
2. Continue for 15 minutes at a challenging to uncomfortable yet manageable pace (RPE 8–9).
3. Cool down for 2–5 minutes at a comfortable pace (RPE 3–4).

Week 4

1. Choose a cardio activity. Take 3–5 minutes to slowly build up to a challenging to an uncomfortable yet manageable pace (RPE 8–9).
2. Continue for 18 minutes at a challenging to uncomfortable yet manageable pace (RPE 8–9).
3. Cool down for 2–5 minutes at a comfortable pace (RPE 3–4).

Core Circuit

Your Core Circuit combines many of the most effective exercises for your abdominals, lower back, and obliques. Benefits include:

- toned midsection
- increased lower back strength and stability
- decreased lower back pain
- improved posture

Note on core work:

It's common to think the abdominal wall is composed of "upper" and "lower" abdominals. Actually, the abdominal wall itself is one muscle called the rectus abdominalis. This muscle is connected to your lower chest on one end and your pelvis on the other. When you think of a "six-pack" you're thinking of the rectus abdominalis. I often get questions about how to tone and flatten the lower section of the abdominal wall, referred to as "lower abs." Here's my take:

Abdominal Exercises

Most abdominal exercises engage the entire abdominal wall. Some are useful in targeting the deep musculature underneath the abdominal wall (transverse abdominalis), and some specifically target the internal/external obliques (sometimes referred to as "love handles"). Abdominal exercises strengthen and develop the abdominal muscles, but play a minor role in burning the pre-existing fat that is covering the abdominals or "belly blankets," as I call them. For this reason, you can train your abdominals consistently and never achieve the toned, flat midsection you may be aiming for.

The take home message is that abdominal exercises are essential to enhancing functional/structural strength and developing the abdominal muscles themselves. However, in order to see the fruits of your labor, you must burn your excess belly blankets. The most effective way to burn belly blankets is through cardiovascular training and nutrition.

Cardiovascular Training

While there is no such thing as spot reduction when it comes to decreasing belly blankets, cardiovascular training helps to utilize stored fat throughout your body. The Cardio-Powervals and Cardio-Rhythm workouts are fabulous ways to help you burn calories, increase your Resting Metabolic Rate (RMR), and metabolize unwanted blankets covering your abdominals.

Nutrition

What you eat plays a leading role in your body's ability to burn belly blankets. If you take in more calories than your body burns, the excess calories are stored as body fat. If you drastically reduce your caloric intake, your metabolism can slow down and your body will use muscle protein for fuel. The key is to develop a way of eating that both fuels your body and supports your intentions. Your Vital Eating Plan in Part III will help you develop a personalized nourishment program that supports a strong, toned core.

Circuit Suggestions:

One to three sets of each exercise is optimal. The key is quality versus quantity. While every exercise has a recommended duration and number of repetitions, make each one your own and challenge yourself. Remember, you want to confuse your body. If you feel you can go longer or do more repetitions with good form (no strain in the neck or lower back), go for it!

I suggest doing 10–25 repetitions. The key is to "feel the burn." If your abdominals do not burn by the fifteenth rep, try working with a more advanced movement. Be sure to choose movements that feel right to you. The only equipment you need is a mat or towel and an optional fit ball.

Abdominal Crunches

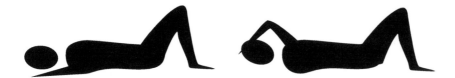

1. Lie on your back with your knees bent, making sure your lower back is pressed firmly to the floor.
2. Place your fingers on your temples with your elbows facing out.
3. Keeping your head in line with your neck, bring your sternum toward your pelvis on a slow 2-count by lifting your shoulders and head off the floor. Come up as far as you can without strain.
4. Slowly exhale as you come up, squeezing your abdominals by pressing your belly button toward your spine. Hold for a slow 2-count, like you're trying to crush a grape with your lower back.
5. Come back to the starting position on a slow 3-count, taking a deep inhalation as you do so.
6. Repeat: up for 2 counts, hold for 2 counts, and then release down for 2 counts.

Note: If you have pain in your neck, I suggest doing the Reverse Crunch.

Reverse Crunch

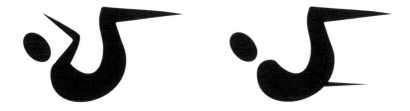

1. Begin in the Abdominal Crunch position.
2. Keep your knees bent and bring them toward your chest, squeezing your abdominals by pressing your belly button toward your spine. Keep your head and neck on the floor throughout the exercise. For added support, place your hands under your gluteus.
3. Slowly lower your legs toward the floor. The range of motion depends on your comfort level. The tension should be in your abdominals.

4. Repeat: up for 2 counts, hold for 2 counts, and then release down for 2 counts. If you feel pain in your lower back, omit this exercise.

Note: An advanced variation of the reverse crunch is the Incline Reverse Crunch.

Boat Pose

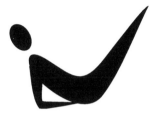

1. Begin by sitting on a mat or towel.
2. Lean back on your forearms.
3. Bring your legs up in the air, creating a V-shape with your upper and lower body.
4. Relax your shoulders and neck as you gaze toward your feet.
5. Hold for 30 seconds to 2 minutes. The key is to "feel the burn."

Note: Where you stop and hold your legs depends on how you feel. If you feel strain in the lower back or neck, bring your legs up to a place where your abdominal muscles contract without strain. You may also decide to place your head on the floor and your hands under your gluteus for added back support. If the discomfort in the back or neck persists, place your heels gently against the wall for added support.

Advanced Variation:

Full Boat Pose
1. Sitting on the floor, bring your legs toward your chest.
2. Tilt your upper body backward so that your lower back carries your weight and your upper back is in a straight line.
3. Extend your arms forward, keeping them parallel to the floor.
4. Stretch your legs and feet together, keeping your back straight.
5. Hold for 15–90 seconds.

For a more advanced variation, I suggest the Full Boat with Fit Ball.

Pilates Reach to Scissor Kick Superset

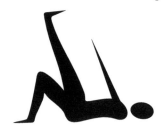

1. Lying on your back, place one leg straight up in the air and plant one leg on the floor in a neutral position. (For an advanced variation, lift and elevate the opposing leg.)
2. Bring your arms up, reaching for your toes. Engage your abdominals by pressing your lower back into the floor.
3. Pulse 10–25 times, keeping your head and neck elevated. Exhale as you reach up and inhale as you lower your torso down.
4. If you feel strain in the neck, omit the pulse and simply hold the contracted up position. If it still feels uncomfortable, omit this movement and proceed to the scissor kicks, keeping your head and neck on the floor.
5. After a 15-second recovery, repeat the pulsing movement with the other leg.
6. At the end of the suggested duration, hold your arms up in the reach position, engaging your abdominals, and perform the scissor kick movement on a 3-count. Inhale and exhale comfortably.

Suggestion: Try 10–25 repetitions for each leg, followed by 10–25 scissor kicks.

Abdominal Bike Ride with Reach

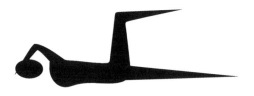

1. Lying on your back, elevate your legs by bringing your knees to your chest.
2. Fully extend your right leg. With your arms extended and hands clasped, reach toward your extended knee. Squeeze your abdominals by exhaling and driving your belly button toward your spine. Picture yourself squeezing a grape with your lower back.

3. Hold this position for a slow 3-count.

4. Release and repeat by straightening your left leg while bringing your right knee to your chest.

Suggestions:

- Try 10–25 repetitions for each side.
- If you experience neck pain, place your head and neck on the floor for the entire movement. Place your hands under your gluteus for added back support and omit the reach with the hands. Experiment with the height of your feet until you find a height that feels right to you.
- For a more advanced movement, add resistance by clasping a light weight with both hands.

Core Hold

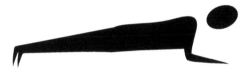

1. Beginning on your stomach, support your weight by lifting up on your forearms and toes.
2. Keep your back flat and your eyes gazing forward.
3. Engage your abdominals by driving your belly button toward your spine.
4. Distribute your weight evenly between your upper and lower body.
5. Hold for 30 seconds to 3 minutes.

Suggestions:

If you need a modification, try elongating your body while keeping your knees on the floor. For a more advanced movement, lift one leg 3–5 inches for 5 seconds to 1 minute, and then switch sides. Finish by holding the original pose with both feet planted.

Yoga Stretch (See page 86–90.)

WORKOUT 3, WEEKS 1–4: LOWER BODY POWER CIRCUIT AND AEROBIC CARDIO

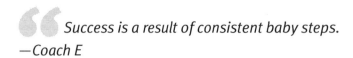 *Success is a result of consistent baby steps.*
—*Coach E*

Warm-Up (See Mental Preparation, Cardio Warm-Up, and Dynamic Stretch, pages 71–75.)

Lower Body Power Circuit

The Lower Body Power Circuit is a high-intensity lower-body circuit that tones, strengthens, and lights your metabolic calorie-burning furnace!

Step-Ups

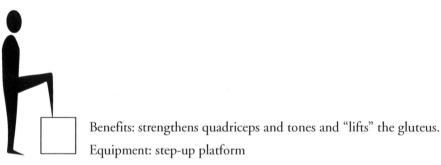

Benefits: strengthens quadriceps and tones and "lifts" the gluteus.

Equipment: step-up platform

1. Place your right foot on a platform. You can use a step, bench, or chair. Choose a height that feels right to you. Keep your upper body still. If you feel as if you're compensating with your upper body, lower the step.
2. Place your left foot 2–3 feet from the step.
3. With your hands on your hips, lift your left knee toward your chest. Do this by both pushing off of your left foot and up with your right leg.
4. Hold this position for a slow 3-count and slowly return to the starting point on a slow 3-count.
5. Repeat. For an added challenge, hold a free weight in each hand while you step up.

Side Step Squats

Benefits: strengthens and tones legs and gluteus.

Equipment: step-up platform

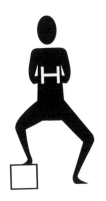

1. Stand parallel to your platform with your right foot planted on the platform and your left foot about two feet away.
2. Inhale and squat down, slightly extending your right knee past 90 degrees. Be mindful not to allow either knee to extend beyond your toes; rotating your hips outward (sticking out your gluteus) helps with this.
3. Exhale and push off of your right leg while raising your left leg out to the side.
4. Repeat 10–15 times with each leg.

Fit Ball Squats

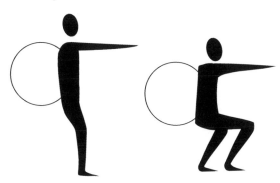

Benefits: strengthens and tones legs and gluteus.

Equipment: fit ball

1. Place your fit ball between the small of your lower back and the wall. If you don't have a fit ball on hand, you can use the wall. If this is uncomfortable, step forward and perform the exercise without the wall or ball. In this case, concentrate on keeping your back straight throughout the movement.
2. Move your legs out two to three feet with legs shoulder-width apart and toes pointed forward. You will feel as if you're leaning back on the ball slightly.
3. Keeping your back straight, inhale and squat down on a slow 3-count by bending at your knees. Break 90 degrees, staying mindful not to allow your knees to go beyond the front of your toes.
4. Hold for a 2-count.
5. Exhale and return to the starting position on a 2-count.
6. Repeat. For added resistance, hold weighted free weights in each hand by your hips.

Fit Ball Inner Thigh Squat

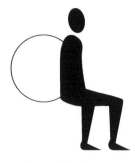

Benefits: strengthens and tones inner thighs and gluteus.

Equipment: fit ball

1. Stand in the same position as the Fit Ball Squat with the exception of your toes. Turn your toes out 3–4 inches, which helps to accentuate the inner thighs.
2. Let your arms hang loosely between your legs.
3. Keeping your back straight, exhale and squat down on a slow 3-count, forming a 90-degree angle at your knees.
4. Hold this position for a slow 3-count.
5. Exhale and slowly stand up on a 2-count.
6. Repeat. Add a free weight for more resistance, if desired.

One-Legged Dead Lift

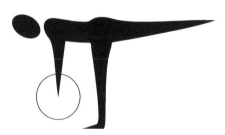

Benefits: increases balance and strengthens and tones hamstrings, gluteus, and the stabilizer muscles of the knee.

1. Anchor your right foot to the floor.
2. With your knee slightly bent, exhale and reach toward the front of your right toe by lifting your left leg behind you. You may do this with or without a free weight in both hands.
3. Hold for a 2-count.
4. Inhale and bring your left foot back to the starting position on a slow 2-count.
5. Complete 10–15 repetitions with each leg.

Lying Fit Ball Hamstring Curl

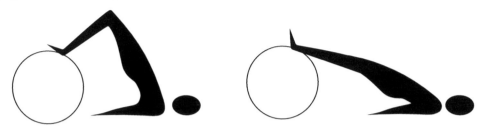

Benefits: strengthens and tones hamstrings, lower back, gluteus, and abdominals.

Equipment: fit ball

1. Lie on your back and place your hands by your hips with your legs outstretched on a fit ball. If you don't have a fit ball, place both feet on the floor with knees 3 inches apart.

2. Lift your pelvis toward the ceiling, engaging your gluteus and lower back. Support your weight with your shoulders and upper back. Be sure to support your head and neck on the floor.

3. Lift your pelvis skyward and, using your feet, exhale and bring your fit ball toward your gluteus, engaging your hamstrings. Hold for a slow 3-count.

4. Inhale and bring the ball back to the starting position, keeping your pelvis elevated for the entire set.

5. Repeat.

One-Legged Pelvic Lift

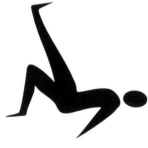

Benefits: tones and strengthens hamstrings and gluteus.

Equipment: fit ball (optional)

1. Lying on your back, place your right foot on the floor and your left foot straight in the air. For a more advanced exercise using the fit ball, place one leg on the fit ball and one leg in the air.

2. Exhale and drive your pelvis toward the sky by pushing off with your right foot, engaging your hamstring and gluteus. Hold for a slow 3-count.

3. Inhale and return to the starting position on a slow 3-count.

4. Repeat 10–15 times with each leg.

Hamstring Curl

Benefits: strengthens and tones hamstrings.

Equipment: ham string curl machine

1. Place the weight pad on the lower third of your calves. Flex your toes. Use a weight that feels challenging but can be done without moving your upper torso for momentum.
2. Exhale and bring the weight pad to your gluteus, engaging your hamstrings. Hold for a slow 2-count.
3. Inhale and lower the weight pad on a slow 3-count.
4. Repeat 10–15 times

Chair Pose

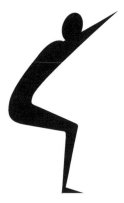

Benefits: strengthens and tones gluteus, quadriceps, and hamstrings.

1. Bend your knees at a 45-degree angle by rotating your pelvis outward as if you are sitting in a chair. Be mindful not to allow your knees to come over your toes.
2. Bring your outstretched arms parallel to your shoulders.
3. Hold this pose and breathe comfortably for 30–90 seconds.

Standing Calf Raises

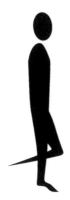

Benefits: strengthens and tones calves.

Equipment: calf machine or platform

1. Use a calf machine or stand at the edge of a stair or step.
2. Let your heels hang off the back of the stair or step.
3. Exhale and stand on your toes, engaging your calves by lifting your heels toward the sky. Hold for a slow 2-count.
4. Inhale and return to the starting position on a slow 3-count.
5. Repeat.

Suggestions:
- For added resistance, hold a free weight in each hand or add weight to the calf machine.
- To vary your workout, try a one-legged calf raise with weight.

After you complete your last circuit, take 2–5 minutes of recovery and proceed to the aerobic cardio portion of your workout. Choose an exercise modality that feels right to you. Some examples include power walking, dancing, running, stationary or outdoor biking, or an elliptical machine.

Aerobic Cardio Set

This segment consists of continuous cardiovascular exercise at a challenging pace (RPE 7–8) for 20–30 minutes. I suggest choosing an intensity that feels less challenging than your Cardio-Powerval and Cardio-Rhythm workouts.

The benefits of aerobic cardio exercise include:
- strengthening your lungs and heart
- increased endurance
- increased fat burning
- decreased anxiety and tension
- increased energy
- increased endorphins

Yoga Stretch (See page 86–90.)

Rest Day/Active Recovery

> ❝ *Life is a process. We are a process. The universe is a process.*
> —*Anne Wilson Schaef*

Rest and active recovery days are essential, regardless of your current fitness level. It's important to note that your body does not transform when you are exercising.

Transformation occurs when you are resting and recovering. The below equation sums up this point:

exercise stimulus + rest = adaptation and transformation

**exercise stimulus + more exercise stimulus without rest =
burnout, physiological plateaus, and injury**

When your inner genius tells you it's time to take a day off from structured training, it's important to listen. Rest days or a cardiovascular recovery workout at a moderate pace (RPE 6) or below allow your body and mind time to recover, repair, and recharge.

Yoga Stretch for Active Recovery or Go with Your Flow! Workouts

Standing Mountain Pose

Benefits: balance, posture, alignment, and stretches entire back.
1. Stand with your feet together and your hands by your side.
2. Raise your toes off the floor, fan them out, and then gently place them back on the floor.

3. Feel how your heels, the outsides of your feet, and the balls of your feet connect with the floor.

4. Tilt your pelvic bone forward.

5. Lift your chest up and out. Roll your shoulders back.

6. Raise the crown of your head toward the ceiling.

7. Inhale and reach your arms to the sky, keeping space between your fingers. Elongate your spine and arms. Feel your body lengthening.

8. Hold this pose for 5 or more breaths.

Standing Side Bend

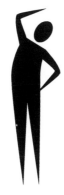

Benefits: increases flexibility in the spine, arms, and rib cage; aligns spinal column; opens lungs to increase oxygen intake.

1. From Mountain Pose, place your right hand on your hip.

2. Raise your left arm straight up, creating a line from your foot to your fingertips.

3. Bend your upper body to the right without forcing the bend. Feel your back and arm muscles stretching.

4. Hold this pose for 5 or more breaths.

5. Repeat on the other side.

Tree Pose

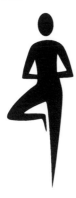

Benefits: increases stability, concentration, and leg strength.

1. Begin by standing with your back straight and your feet shoulder-width apart.

2. Mentally "anchor" your left foot to the earth.

3. Fix your gaze on a specific spot in front of you.
4. Lift your right foot and place it on your left inner thigh, above or below your knee.
5. Work to turn your right knee out at a 90-degree angle by opening your pelvis.
6. Place your hands together over your heart.
7. Hold for 5 or more breaths.
8. Repeat on the other side.

Note: If you have difficulty with balance, place one hand on a wall for added support.

Standing Forward Fold

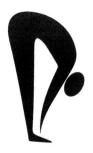

Benefits: stretches hamstrings, calves, and hips.
1. Begin by establishing a smooth flowing breath by breathing from your abdomen, in through your nose and out through your mouth.
2. Stand with your feet hip-width apart.
3. Using your hips as a hinge, fold forward by allowing your upper body to fall toward the earth.
4. Bend your knees to take pressure off your lower back.
5. Clasp your elbows with opposite hands.
6. Breath comfortably, letting gravity pull you downward.
7. Gently sway from side to side.
8. Hold in the center for 5 or more breaths.

Warrior I

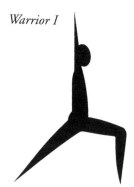

Benefits: enhances balance, concentration, and flexibility; tones and strengthens legs, groin, chest, and shoulders.

1. Stand with your feet together and step forward with your right foot about 3–4 feet.

2. Bend your right knee so that it is in line with your right ankle.

3. Turn your left foot out 45 degrees.

4. Align your left ankle with your right ankle.

5. Draw your right hip back and your left hip forward, so that your hips are square. Distribute your weight to your front leg.

6. Bring your arms out to the side and up over your head.

7. Bring your hands together over your head with palms touching.

8. Look up at your thumbs.

9. Tilt back slightly as if you are about to do a backbend. You should feel a stretch in your lower back.

10. Slide your shoulder blades down your back, opening your chest.

11. Hold this position for 5 or more breaths.

12. Repeat on the other side.

Warrior II

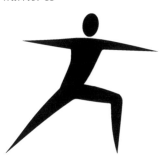

Benefits: enhances balance, concentration, flexibility, and strength; tones legs, groin, chest, and shoulders.

1. From Warrior I, with your right leg in front, bring your arms down so that they are parallel to the floor.

2. Point your right arm forward and your left arm behind you, keeping your shoulder blades wide and your palms facing down.

3. Bring your shoulders over your hips and look over your front hand, keeping your head in a comfortable position.

4. Hold this position for 5 or more breaths.

5. Repeat on the other side.

Warrior III

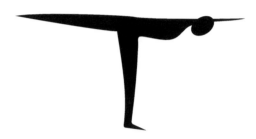

Benefits: enhances balance, concentration, flexibility, and strength; tones legs, core, and arms.

1. From Warrior I, with your right leg in front, place your hands on your hips.
2. Bring your weight forward onto your right foot as you raise your left leg straight behind you.
3. Bring your torso forward until it's parallel to the floor.
4. Keep your neck aligned with the natural extension of your body and your eyes looking toward the front of your toe.
5. Flex your raised foot and engage the muscles of your raised leg.
6. Bring your arms along the sides of your body or parallel to the sides of your head.
7. Hold for 5 or more breaths.
8. Repeat on the other side.

Downward Dog

Benefits: stretches and strengthens your whole body and helps relieve lower back pain.

1. Begin on your hands and knees with your wrists under your shoulders and your knees under your hips.
2. Exhale and lift your tail up by straightening your legs and keeping a slight bend at your knees.
3. Press your heels toward the floor. Distribute your weight to your legs by pushing off with your fingers and palms.

4. Let your head hang naturally. Spread your shoulder blades away from your ears, opening up your collarbone.

5. Hold for 5 or more breaths.

Cobra

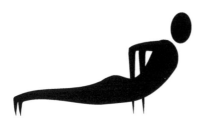

Benefits: stretches back muscles, abdomen, and upper body.

1. Begin by lying on your stomach.

2. Place your hands on the floor, parallel to your pectoral muscles.

3. Keep your toes pointed with the tops of your toes on the floor.

4. Inhale and slide your chest forward, keeping your hands in the same position.

5. Roll your shoulders back and lift your chest higher, keeping your lower ribs on the floor and your neck in a neutral position.

6. Hold for 5 or more breaths.

Suggestion: Straighten your arms, and gently lift your pelvis and quadriceps off the floor into Upward Facing Dog for a more advanced stretch.

Locust Pose

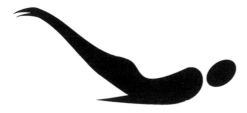

Benefits: enhances strength in your upper legs and lower back and stretches your lower back and abdominal wall.

1. Lie on your stomach with your forehead on the floor.
2. Slide your hands under your thighs with your palms up. If this feels uncomfortable, place your hands by the sides of your hips with your palms up.
3. Inhale deeply and raise your head, legs, and chest in the air as far as it feels comfortable to you.
4. Hold this pose for 5 or more breaths.

Child's Pose

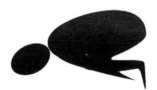

Benefits: gently stretches hips, thighs, and ankles; helps relieve stress, fatigue, and back pain.

Equipment: yoga block, pillow, or towel (optional)

1. Kneel on the floor and sit on your feet with your heels facing out.
2. Separate your knees hip-width distance. If this is uncomfortable, place a folded towel, yoga block, or pillow under your tailbone for added support.
3. Gently lean forward and place your forehead on the floor.
4. Rest your arms along your torso, palms facing up.
5. Press your tailbone toward your feet, gently stretching your lower back.
6. Hold this pose for 5 or more breaths.

Cobbler's Pose

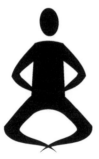

Benefits: stretches and opens hips and groin.

1. Sit on the floor with the bottoms of your feet touching and your knees pointed outward. Hold your feet.
2. Keeping your spine long, gently press your knees toward the floor.
3. Hold for 5 or more breaths.

Head to Knee

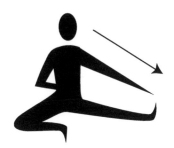

Benefits: stretches hamstrings.
1. Sit with legs fully extended in front of you.
2. Bring the sole of your right foot to the inside of your left thigh.
3. Square your torso over your extended left leg.
4. Begin to bend forward, keeping your back from rounding by bringing your heart toward your left knee while lengthening your spine.
5. Keep your left foot flexed while pressing your left thigh to the floor.
6. Bend as far as you feel comfortable. You may decide to hold on to your extended leg or place your hands on the floor.
7. Hold for 5 or more breaths.
8. Repeat with your right foot extended.

Happy Baby Pose

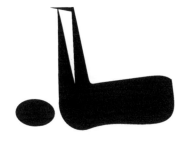

Benefits: stretches lower back and upper thighs.

1. Lie on your back.
2. Bring your legs up to your hips, knees bent.
3. Clasp your hands on the tops of your shins or feet and bring your knees toward your shoulders.
4. Pull your knees closer, feeling the stretch in your lower back.
5. Hold for 5 or more breaths.

Lying Side Fold

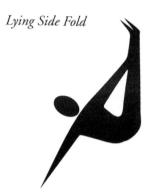

Benefits: stretches lower back.

1. From Happy Baby, bring both legs to your right side, keeping your shoulders on the floor. Turn your head away from your knees.
2. Hold for 5 or more breaths.
3. Repeat on the left side.

Bridge Pose

Benefits: stretches and strengthens lower back.

1. Lie on your back and bend your knees with your feet on the floor.
2. Press your feet into the floor, driving your pelvis toward the sky.
3. Clasp your hands under your buttocks and pull them down toward your feet.
4. Lift your chin and press the top of your sternum toward your chin.
5. Hold for 5 or more breaths.

Dog-Cat

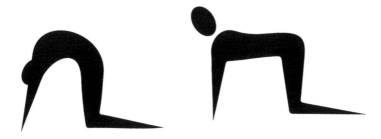

Benefits: stretches back, arms, shoulders, hips, heels, and hamstrings; opens chest.

1. Begin on your hands and knees with your wrists under your shoulders and your knees under your hips.
2. Keep your back flat and parallel to the floor. Gaze at the floor.
3. Press down on your hands, lift your tailbone, arch your back, and stretch your head toward the ceiling.
4. Hold for 5 or more breaths.
5. When you feel ready, go into "cat tilt" by pulling your abdominals toward your spine, tucking your tailbone up and under, and rounding your back.
6. Gently drop your head downward and gaze at the floor between your knees.
7. Hold for 5 or more breaths.
8. Repeat several times.

Bird-Dog

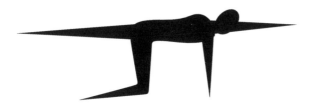

Benefits: stretches and strengthens abdominals, lower back, arms, and legs.

1. From Dog-Cat, return to a neutral position and bring your right arm straight out so that it is parallel to your ear.
2. Bring your left leg straight back, aligning your leg with your hips and outstretched arm.
3. Engage your abdominals, lower back, and gluteus. Focus your gaze toward your outstretched arm.

4. Hold for 5 or more breaths.

5. Repeat on the other side.

Modified Bow Pose

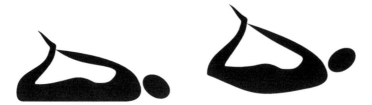

Benefits: increases flexibility in the quadriceps and strengthens knees.

Equipment: stretching cord or towel (optional)

1. Lie on your stomach and rest your head to one side.

2. Bend your left knee and grip your left ankle with your left hand.

3. Bend your right knee and grip your right ankle with your right hand. If this is uncomfortable for you, use a stretching cord or towel.

4. Hold for 5 or more breaths.

Modified Pigeon Pose

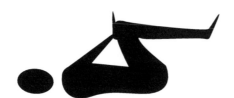

Benefits: Stretches gluteus, hip joint, and muscles connecting to the lower back.

1. Lie down on your back and bend your knees with your feet on the floor.

2. Cross your right leg over your left so your right ankle rests just below your left knee.

3. Hold your left thigh with both hands and gently pull your leg toward you until you feel a stretch in your right gluteus and outer thigh.

4. Hold for 5 or more breaths.

5. Repeat with your other leg.

Hero Pose and Triceps Stretch

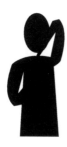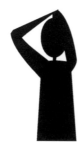

Benefits: stretches triceps, shoulders, hips, knees, thighs, and groin.

1. Begin by kneeling on the floor with your knees touching.
2. Bring your heels out along the sides of your buttocks.
3. Keeping your back straight, bring your buttocks to the floor between your legs.
4. Raise your right arm straight in the air and bend your forearm, leaving your elbow straight in the air and your hand on your upper back.
5. Use your left hand to stretch your right triceps by gently pressing down on your right elbow.
6. Hold for 5 or more breaths.
7. Repeat with the other arm.

Cleansing Breaths

Benefits: a relaxing way to bring your workout to a close.

1. Begin in Mountain Pose.
2. Exhale and swan dive down toward the floor, bending at your waist. Allow your knees to bend so that you're not putting pressure on your lower back.
3. Inhale and sweep your arms back up as you return to Mountain Pose.
4. Repeat for 5 or more breaths.

WORKOUT 4, WEEKS 1–4: CARDIO-POWERVALS AND CORE CIRCUIT

Practice yourself, for heaven's sake in little things, and then proceed to greater. — Epictetus

The Cardio-Powervals workout on this day consists of a series of intervals lasting three minutes and is designed to maximize physiological adaptation and caloric burn. As always, choose the type of exercise and the intensity that feels right to you. The estimated intensity that corresponds to a challenging pace (RPE 8) during a short Powerval (30–90 seconds) is often higher than that of a RPE of 8 during a 3-minute Powerval. Customize the workout intensity and duration to fit your needs.

Warm-Up (See Mental Preparation, Cardio Warm-Up, and Dynamic Stretch, pages 71–75.)

Cardio-Powervals

Week 1

1. Choose a cardio activity. Then complete 3 x 3-minute Powervals at a challenging to very challenging pace (RPE 7–8.5). Follow each Powerval with a 2-minute recovery at a moderate pace (RPE 4–5).
2. After completing all three Powervals, cool down for 2–5 minutes at a comfortable pace (RPE 3–4).

Week 2

1. Choose a cardio activity. Then complete 4 x 3-minute Powervals at a challenging to a very challenging pace (RPE 7–8.5). Follow each Powerval with a 2-minute recovery at a moderate pace (RPE 4–5).
2. Cool down for 2–5 minutes at a comfortable pace (RPE 3–4).

Week 3

1. Choose a cardio activity. Then complete 5 x 3-minute Powervals at a challenging to a very challenging pace (RPE 7–8.5). Follow each Powerval with a 2-minute recovery at a moderate pace (RPE 4–5).
2. Cool down for 2–5 minutes at a comfortable pace (RPE 3–4).

Week 4

1. Choose a cardio activity. Then complete 6 x 3-minute Powervals at a challenging to very challenging pace (RPE 7–8.5). Follow each Powerval with a 2-minute recovery at a moderate pace (RPE 4–5).
2. Cool down for 2–5 minutes at a comfortable pace (RPE 3–4).

Notes: If you're relatively new to exercise or coming off of a significant hiatus, choose a moderately challenging pace in the RPE 7–7.5 range. If you've been exercising consistently for a while, I suggest pushing your pace to an RPE 8.5–9 range or a very challenging to an uncomfortable yet manageable pace.

Core Circuit

Modified/Full Boat Pose to Scissors Kick Superset

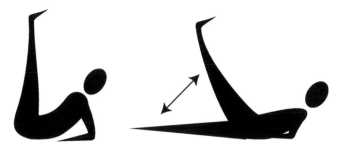

1. Begin in the boat position that feels right to you. (See page 95 for a full description.) Hold for 30–60 seconds.
2. Slowly lift your legs up and down in a scissor-like motion.
3. Use an extension that feels right for you. The tension should be on the abdominals, not the lower back.
4. Do 10–25 scissor kicks with each leg.

For an advanced version, cradle a fit ball between your legs while doing the lift.

Jackknife/Fit Ball Exchange

1. Begin by lying on your back with your legs in an L-position.
2. If you have a fit ball, hold it with outstretched arms behind your head.
3. Reach up and place the ball between your legs. Be sure to squeeze your abdominals by pressing your belly button toward your spine.

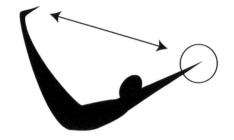

4. Keeping your arms extended and abdominals squeezed, slowly bring your legs toward the floor. Lower your legs as far as you feel comfortable without touching the floor. Hold for a slow 3-count.

5. Bring the ball back up to your hands. Hold for a slow 3-count.

6. Bring the ball back behind your head to the start position.

7. Repeat 10–25 times.

Seated Trunk Twist

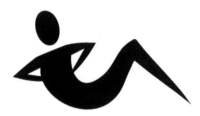

1. Sit on the floor with your feet planted in front of you, balancing on your gluteus.

2. Turning your head and keeping your hands clasped, twist from right to left, tapping the floor with your fingers.

3. Repeat 10–25 times on each side.

Suggestions:

- Customize by elevating and crossing your feet.
- Hold a free weight in your hands for added resistance.

Abdominal Rope Climb

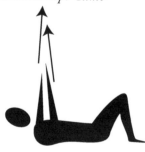

1. Lie on your back with your legs in an L-position.

2. Imagine a rope hanging from the ceiling.

3. "Climb the rope," reaching right over left for 2–3 pulls. Squeeze your abdominals by pressing your belly button toward your spine.

4. Hold for a slow 3-count and release by slowly "climbing down the rope."

5. Repeat 10–25 times.

Yoga Stretch (See page 86–90.)

Bonus Workout: Go with Your Flow!

> " *Happy are those who dream dreams and are ready to pay the price to make those dreams come true.* —Leon Joseph Cardinal Suenens

The Go with Your Flow! bonus session is an opportunity to integrate other activities you enjoy into your program. The idea is not to choose the "right" workout, but a workout that feels good to you. In fact, it doesn't have to be a workout at all—enjoy means to be in-joy! Ask yourself, *How would I like to celebrate my mental and physical being today?*

Perhaps you would enjoy a hike? A game of tennis? An exercise class? A yoga stretch? An endurance bike ride or run? A long walk with a friend? One of my favorite things to do with my wife, Theresa, and our two-year-old daughter, Bianca, is to have a dance party in our living room. I invite you to think of this session as a way to feel vibrant and alive in the present moment!

Suggestions:

- Think about moving without expectations or judgment. In other words, think about moving to move, as opposed to how well you do it. Notice how liberating this feels.
- I invite you not to wear a watch. Stop at some point and be grateful for the ability to move and for the brilliance of being alive!
- Enjoy! And don't take yourself too seriously!

Weeks 5–8 Workouts at a Glance

Day	Warm-Up	Workout	Stretch
Monday	Mental Preparation Cardio (5–15 min.) Dynamic Stretch Power March Shoulder Circles Arm Circles Standing Trunk Twist Hip Circles Half Squat Leg Swing	Plyo-Pump Circuit 2 x 1-2 min. line drill or toe tap 2 x 1-2 min. earth-sky jumps or earth-sky without jump 2 x 1-2 min. scissor jumps or scissor taps 2 x 1-2 min. inner and outer thigh cross or taps 2 x 1-2 min. jump rope (with or without rope and jump) 2 x 1-2 min. stair climbers or stair taps 2 x 1-2 min. squat-thrust-jump or squat-extend-stand 2 x 1-2 min. foot fire or power march 2 x 1-2 min. step jumps or step taps Cardio-Powervals Week 5: 5 x 1 min. at a challenging to uncomfortable yet manageable pace (RPE 7–9). Follow each with a 1-min. recovery at a moderate pace (RPE 4–5) Week 6: 6 x 1 min. at a challenging to uncomfortable yet manageable pace (RPE 7–9). Follow each with a 1-min. recovery at a moderate pace (RPE 4–5) Week 7: 10 x 45 sec. at a challenging to uncomfortable yet manageable pace (RPE 7–9). Follow each with a 30-sec. recovery at a moderate pace (RPE 4–5) Week 8: 7 x 1 min. at a challenging to uncomfortable yet manageable pace (RPE 7–9). Follow each with a 1-min. recovery at a moderate pace (RPE 4–5) Cool down 2–5 min. at a comfortable pace (RPE 3–4)	Yoga Stretch Standing Mountain Pose Standing Side Bend Downward Dog Cobra Modified Pigeon Pose Bridge Pose Happy Baby Pose Cleansing Breaths
Tuesday	Mental Preparation Cardio (5–15 min.) Dynamic Stretch Power March Shoulder Circles Arm Circles Standing Trunk Twist Hip Circles Half Squat Leg Swing	Cardio-Rhythm 3–5 min. build to a very challenging to uncomfortable yet manageable pace (RPE 8–9) Week 5: 20 min. at a very challenging to uncomfortable yet manageable pace (RPE 8–9) Week 6: 3 x 8 min. at a very challenging to uncomfortable yet manageable pace (RPE 8–9) Week 7: 26 min. at a very challenging to uncomfortable yet manageable pace (RPE 8–9) Week 8: 6 x 5 min. at a very challenging to uncomfortable yet manageable pace (RPE 8–9) Cool down 3–5 min. at a comfortable pace (RPE 3–4) Core Circuit 2 x 10–25 abdominal crunches 2 x 1 min. boat pose (modified or full) 2 x 10–25 reps. Pilates reach to scissor superset 2 x 10–25 reps. abdominal bike ride with reach 2 x 30 sec.–2 min. core hold	Yoga Stretch Standing Mountain Pose Standing Side Bend Downward Dog Cobra Modified Pigeon Pose Bridge Pose Happy Baby Pose Cleansing Breaths

Wednesday	Mental Preparation Cardio (5–15 min.) Dynamic Stretch Power March Shoulder Circles Arm Circles Standing Trunk Twist Hip Circles Half Squat Leg Swing	**Fit Fusion Circuit** 2 x 10–15 reps. incline chest press 2 x 30 sec. plank to push-up superset 2 x 10–15 reps. squat/hammer curl/press superset **Cardio-Powervals** 2-min. warm-up at a moderate pace (RPE 5–6) 3 x 75 sec. at a challenging to an uncomfortable yet manageable pace (RPE 8–9). Follow each with a 45-sec. recovery at a moderate pace (RPE 5) **Fit Fusion Circuit** 2 x 10–15 reps. fit ball inner thigh squat 2 x 1 min. boat pose (modified or full) 2 x 10–25 reps. abdominal bike ride with reach 2 x 1–2 min. earth-sky jumps 2 x 1–2 min. scissor jumps **Cardio-Powervals** 2-min. warm-up at a moderate pace (RPE 5–6) 3 x 75 sec. at a challenging to an uncomfortable yet manageable pace (RPE 8–9). Follow each with a 45-sec. recovery at a moderate pace (RPE 5) **Fit Fusion Circuit** 2 x 10–15 step-ups 2 x 10–15 side step squats 2 x 10–15 triceps dips	**Yoga Stretch** Standing Mountain Pose Standing Side Bend Downward Dog Cobra Modified Pigeon Pose Bridge Pose Happy Baby Pose Cleansing Breaths
Thursday	Rest or Active Recovery Day		
Friday	Mental Preparation Cardio (5–15 min.) Dynamic Stretch Power March Shoulder Circles Arm Circles Standing Trunk Twist Hip Circles Half Squat Leg Swing	**Cardio-Ladder** **Week 5:** 2 min. at a moderate pace (RPE 6) 2 min. at a challenging pace (RPE 7) 2 min. at a very challenging pace (RPE 8) 2 min. at an uncomfortable yet manageable pace (RPE 9) Repeat ladder 2–3 times. **Week 6:** 3 min. at a moderate pace (RPE 6) 3 min. at a very challenging pace (RPE 8) 3 min. at an uncomfortable yet manageable pace (RPE 9) Repeat ladder 2–3 times. **Week 7:** 3 min. at a moderate pace (RPE 6) 4 min. at a very challenging pace (RPE 8) 4 min. at a bit more than a very challenging pace (RPE 8.5) 4 min. at an uncomfortable yet manageable pace (RPE 9) Repeat ladder 2–3 times. **Week 8:** 5 min. at a challenging pace (RPE 7) 5 min. at a very challenging pace (RPE 8) 5 min. at an uncomfortable yet manageable pace (RPE 9) Repeat ladder 2–3 times. Cool down 2–5 min. at a comfortable pace (RPE 3–4)	**Yoga Stretch** Standing Mountain Pose Standing Side Bend Downward Dog Cobra Modified Pigeon Pose Bridge Pose Happy Baby Pose Cleansing Breaths
Saturday	Go with Your Flow!		
Sunday	Rest or Active Recovery Day		

Weeks 5–8 Workout Descriptions

WORKOUT 1, WEEKS 5–8: PLYO-PUMP CIRCUIT AND CARDIO-POWERVALS

> *What the caterpillar calls the end of the world, the master calls a butterfly.* — *Richard Bach*

Plyo-Pump is a heart pumping, endorphin-filled circuit designed to burn calories while toning and strengthening your entire body. This workout is based on the science of plyometrics and power training. Plyometrics are short, explosive movements such as jumping and skipping that involve powerful muscular contractions in response to rapid stretching of the involved muscles.

The Plyo-Pump Circuit workout can:

- enhance muscle confusion (often leading to enhanced physiological adaptation)
- increase strength and power
- increase balance and agility
- increase caloric burn

Warm-Up (See Mental Preparation, Cardio Warm-Up, and Dynamic Stretch, pages 71–75.)

Plyo-Pump Circuit

Note: Plyometric/Power Training is an intermediate to advanced training modality. If you have any prohibitive injuries, I suggest the non-impact version of each exercise.

Suggestions:

- Shoot for 1–2 minutes at each exercise. Take a 1-minute recovery before beginning the next exercise.
- Do 1–3 sets of the entire circuit. (1 set = completion of each exercise.)
- Take 1–2 minutes recovery after each set.
- Take 2–3 minutes recovery before beginning your Powervals.

Line Drill

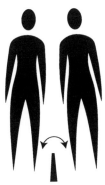

Benefits: caloric burn; tones and strengthens legs and gluteus.

Equipment: platform

1. Place a 2- to 3-foot piece of string on the floor, draw an imaginary line, or stand next to a platform or step.
2. Standing parallel to your line or step, bend your knees slightly. Lock your hands in front of your chest and jump laterally over your step, keeping your feet together.
3. After you land, immediately jump back to the other side of the rope or step.
4. Repeat.

Non-impact suggestion:

Toe-Tap

1. Instead of jumping, quickly tap your left foot to your right foot.
2. Repeat the process with your right foot.
3. Perform the toe tap at a fast tempo, maintaining a straight back.

Earth-Sky Jumps

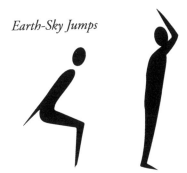

Benefits: caloric burn; tones and strengthens legs and gluteus.

1. From a standing position, squat down and touch your knees, ankles, or the floor with your hands.
2. Jump up, reaching for the sky.
3. Repeat while maintaining a steady tempo.

Non-impact suggestion:

Earth-Sky Without Jump

Instead of jumping off the floor, stand straight up and reach for the sky.

Advanced suggestion:

Weighted Earth-Sky

Add 3- to 10-pound free weights for extra resistance.

Scissor Jumps

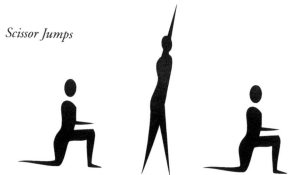

Benefits: caloric burn; tones and strengthens legs, gluteus, and arms.

1. Take a large step forward with your right leg.
2. Place your arms straight over your head.
3. Jump in the air in a scissor motion, switching the position of your right and left leg.
4. After you land, repeat to create a continuous scissor motion.

Non-impact suggestion:

Scissor Taps

Scissor your feet quickly and continuously without jumping.

Advanced suggestion:

Weighted Scissor Jumps

Add 3- to 10-pound free weights.

Inner and Outer Thigh Cross

Benefits: caloric burn; tones and strengthens inner/outer thighs and gluteus.

1. Jump up and extend your legs out to the side.
2. Upon landing, jump up again and cross your left leg over your right.
3. Immediately jump back to the outward position.

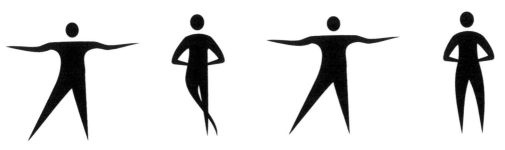

4. Repeat, leading with the right leg.
5. Alternate legs in a continuous crossing motion.

Non-impact suggestion:

Inner Thigh Taps

Instead of jumping, alternate crossing your legs and tapping your feet.

Jump Rope

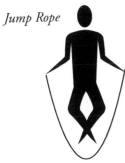

Benefits: caloric burn; tones and strengthens legs, gluteus, and arms.

Equipment: jump rope (optional)

1. With or without a rope, begin to jump in place, keeping your feet together with a slight bend at your knees.
2. Maintain a steady tempo. If you are not using a rope, remember to rotate your arms in small, fast circles as if you were actually jumping over a rope.

Non-impact suggestion:

Mirror the jump rope movement without a rope and without leaving the floor. Instead, turn the imaginary rope over by rotating your hands and simultaneously lifting your heels by shifting your weight to your toes.

Advanced suggestions:

One-Legged Jumping

Jump rope keeping one foot off of the floor.

Increased Tempo

Speed up the tempo of both your hand turnovers and your jumps.

Stair Climbers

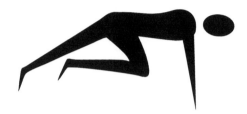

Benefits: caloric burn; tones and strengthens legs, gluteus, arms, and abdominals.

1. Begin on your hands and toes. Lift your right knee toward your chest, keeping your left foot planted.
2. Bring your right leg back to the starting position while simultaneously driving your left knee toward your chest, as if you were running in place.
3. Repeat in a continuous motion, maintaining a steady tempo while keeping your back as still as possible.

Non-impact suggestion:

Stair Taps

1. Instead of the running motion, pick up your right foot and bring your knee toward your chest.
2. Tap your foot on the floor as you reach the closest point between your knee and chest.
3. Bring your foot back to the starting position before beginning the same movement with the other foot.

Squat-Thrust-Jump

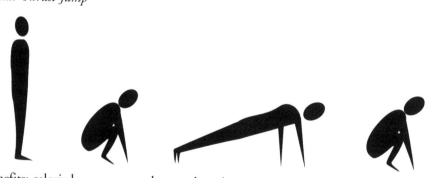

Benefits: caloric burn; tones and strengthens legs, gluteus, arms, and abdominals.

1. Squat and place your hands on the floor, just below your chest and shoulder-width apart.
2. Thrust both feet back, landing on your toes while extending your entire body. Keep your legs straight and your back flat.
3. Immediately jump back, landing with your feet close to your hands.
4. Explode upward, jumping off the floor and fully extending your legs. Thrust your hands skyward.
5. Land and repeat in a continuous, brisk motion.

Non-impact suggestion:

Squat-Extend-Stand
1. Instead of thrusting back, step back leading with your right leg, followed by your left.
2. Step forward the same way.
3. Stand straight up.
4. Squat down and repeat in a continuous, brisk motion.

Foot Fire

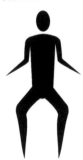

Benefits: caloric burn; strengthens and tones legs and gluteus.
1. Squat down, creating a 120-degree angle at your knees.
2. Place your arms out, palms up.
3. Alternate lifting your right and left foot 1–2 inches off the floor as fast as you can in a continuous, explosive motion.
4. Keep your upper body as still as possible and seek to hold your squat for the entire set.

Non-impact suggestion:

Power March
1. Stand and clasp your hands together with your elbows pointing out. Keep your clasped hands just below your collarbone for the entire set.

2. Drive your right knee up toward your clasped hands. The intention is to hit your hands with your knee. If you can't touch your knee to your hand, that's okay. Do what feels comfortable.
3. Repeat with your left knee.
4. Continue for 1–2 minutes.

Step Jumps

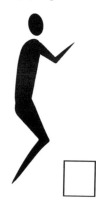

Benefits: caloric burn; strengthens and tones legs and gluteus.

Equipment: platform or step

1. Set your step to a height that feels challenging yet doable for the full set.
2. Stand 2 feet from the step.
3. Squat down and bring your elbows back.
4. Explode onto the step, jumping off of both feet and thrusting your arms forward.
5. Step down slowly, ready yourself, and repeat.

Non-impact suggestion:

Step Taps

1. Step up with your right foot as if you were climbing a stair. If possible, adjust the height to fit your needs.
2. Keeping your foot planted, step up with the other foot.
3. Step down and repeat.

Cardio-Powervals

Week 5

1. Choose a cardio activity. Then complete 5 x 1-minute Powervals at a challenging to an uncomfortable yet manageable pace (RPE 7–9). Follow each Powerval with a 1-minute recovery at a moderate pace (RPE 4–5).
2. After completing all five Powervals, cool down for 2–5 minutes at a comfortable pace (RPE 3–4).

Week 6

1. Choose a cardio activity. Then complete 6 x 1-minute Powervals at a challenging to an

uncomfortable yet manageable pace (RPE 7–9). Follow each Powerval with a 1-minute recovery at a moderate pace (RPE 4–5).

2. After completing all five Powervals, cool down for 2–5 minutes at a comfortable pace (RPE 3–4).

Week 7

1. Choose a cardio activity. Then complete 10 x 45-second Powervals at a challenging to an uncomfortable yet manageable pace (RPE 7–9). Follow each Powerval with a 30-second recovery at a moderate pace (RPE 4–5).

2. Cool down for 2–5 minutes at a comfortable pace (RPE 3–4).

Week 8

1. Choose a cardio activity. Then complete 7 x 1-minute Powervals at a challenging to uncomfortable yet manageable pace (RPE 7–9). Follow each Powerval with a 1-minute recovery at a moderate pace (RPE 4–5).

2. After completing all five Powervals, cool down for 2–5 minutes at a comfortable pace (RPE 3–4).

Yoga Stretch (See page 86–90.)

WORKOUT 2, WEEKS 5–8: CARDIO-RHYTHM AND CORE CIRCUIT

Skill to do comes from doing.
—Ralph Waldo Emerson

Warm-Up (See Mental Preparation, Cardio Warm-Up, and Dynamic Stretch, pages 71–75.)

Cardio-Rhythm

Week 5

1. Choose a cardio activity. Take 3–5 minutes to slowly build up to a very challenging to an uncomfortable yet manageable pace (RPE 8–9).
2. Continue for 20 minutes at a very challenging to an uncomfortable yet manageable pace (RPE 8–9).
3. Cool down for 2–5 minutes at a comfortable pace (RPE 3–4).

Week 6

1. Choose a cardio activity. Take 3–5 minutes to slowly build up to a very challenging to an uncomfortable yet manageable pace (RPE 8–9).
2. Complete 3 x 8-minute intervals at a very challenging to an uncomfortable yet manageable pace (RPE 8–9). Follow each Powerval with a 3-minute recovery at a moderate pace (RPE 4–5).
3. Cool down for 2–5 minutes at a comfortable pace (RPE 3–4).

Week 7

1. Choose a cardio activity. Take 3–5 minutes to slowly build up to a very challenging to uncomfortable yet manageable pace (RPE 8–9).
2. Continue for 26 minutes at a very challenging to uncomfortable yet manageable pace (RPE 8–9).
3. Cool down for 2–5 minutes at a comfortable pace (RPE 3–4).

Week 8

1. Choose a cardio activity. Take 3–5 minutes to slowly build up to a very challenging to uncomfortable yet manageable pace (RPE 8–9).

2. Complete 6 x 5-minute intervals at a very challenging to an uncomfortable yet manageable pace (RPE 8–9). Follow each Powerval with a 5-minute recovery at a moderate pace (RPE 4–5).

3. Cool down for 2–5 minutes at a comfortable pace (RPE 3–4).

Core Circuit

2 x 10–25 *Abdominal Crunches* (See description on page 94.)

2 x 1 min. *Boat Pose* (See description on page 95.)

2 x 10–25 reps. *Pilates Reach to Scissor Kick Superset* (See description on page 96.)

2 x 10–25 reps. *Abdominal Bike Ride with Reach* (See description on pages 96–97.)

2 x 30 sec.–3 min. *Core Hold* (See description on page 97.)

Yoga Stretch (See pages 86–90.)

WORKOUT 3, WEEKS 5–8: FIT FUSION CIRCUIT

> ❝ *An inspired purpose put into action can move mountains.*
> *—Coach E*

The Fit Fusion Circuit is an integration of key exercises from past workouts, new dynamic movements, and high-intensity Cardio-Powervals. I suggest that you complete 1–3 sets of each exercise and allow yourself 30–60 seconds of recovery between exercises. The result is a super-effective, full body fitness blast!

Warm-Up (See Mental Preparation, Cardio Warm-Up, and Dynamic Stretch, pages 71–75.)

Fit Fusion Circuit

Incline Chest Press (See description on pages 75–76.)

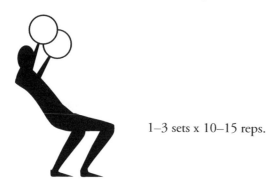

1–3 sets x 10–15 reps.

Plank to Push-Up Superset

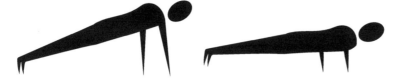

Benefits: strengthens and tones the entire body, with an emphasis on core, arms, and chest.

Equipment: mat or towel

1. Place your hands shoulder-width apart on the floor or mat.
2. Press down with your forearms and hands and lift up on your toes.

3. Be mindful not to let your chest sink. Press back through your heels, creating a straight line from your shoulders to your hips.

4. Hold this plank position for 30 seconds.

5. Proceed into a slow push-up, inhaling and lowering your body down on a slow 5-count, keeping your elbows tight to your rib cage.

6. Hold the low push-up for a slow 3-count.

7. Exhale and explode up on a 2-count.

8. Complete 5 repetitions of the slow push-up before returning to the plank hold for another 30–40 seconds. I suggest doing three rounds of the plank hold with three slow push-ups for each set.

Note: See page 77 for push-up modifications.

Squat/Hammer Curl/Press Superset

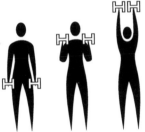

Benefits: strengthens and tones total body, with an emphasis on arms, legs, gluteus, and core.

Equipment: free weights

1. Begin by standing with your hands comfortably by your sides.

2. Slowly squat down using a chair or bench to ensure your knees do not pass the front of your toes.

3. As you slowly stand back up, perform a hammer curl by bringing the sides of your wrists toward your shoulders while keeping your elbows tight to your rib cage.

4. From this position slowly press your hands skyward, finishing above the crown of your head.

5. Reverse direction by slowly bringing your fists down to shoulder level and then back to the starting position.

6. Repeat.

Cardio-Powervals

1. Choose an exercise that feels good to you: treadmill, stationary bike, power march, etc.

2. Start with a 2-minute warm-up at a moderate intensity (RPE 5–6).

3. Then complete 3 x 75-second Powervals at a challenging to an uncomfortable yet manageable pace (RPE 8–9). Follow each Powerval with a 45-second recovery at a moderate pace (RPE 5).

Fit Fusion Circuit

Fit Ball Inner Thigh Squat (See description on page 100.)
1–3 sets x 10–15 reps.

Boat Pose (See description on page 95.)
1–3 sets x 1 min.

Abdominal Bike Ride with Reach (See description on pages 96–97.)
1–3 sets x 10–25 reps.

Earth-Sky Jumps (See description on page 123.)
1–3 sets x 1–2 min.

Scissor Jumps (See description on page 124.)
1–3 sets x 1–2 min.

Cardio-Powervals

1. Choose a cardio activity. Start with a 2-minute warm-up at a moderate pace (RPE 5–6).
2. Then complete 3 x 75-second Powervals at a challenging to an uncomfortable yet manageable pace (RPE 8–9). Follow each Powerval with a 30-second recovery at a moderate pace (RPE 5).

Fit Fusion Circuit

Step-Ups (See description on page 98.)
1–3 sets x 10–15 reps.

Side Step Squats (See description on pages 98–99.)
1–3 sets x 10–15 reps.

Triceps Dips (See description on page 80.)
1–3 sets x 10–15 reps.

Yoga Stretch (See page 86.)

WORKOUT 4, WEEKS 5–8: CARDIO-LADDER

> *When you discover your mission, you will feel its demand.*
> *It will fill you with enthusiasm and burning desire to get to work on it.*
> *— W. Clement Stone*

This workout is designed to keep your body guessing and adapting by consistently increasing and decreasing your intensity (RPE) during the main set. I call this "climbing the ladder."

Warm-Up (See Mental Preparation, Cardio Warm-Up, and Dynamic Stretch, pages 71–75.)

Cardio-Ladder

Week 5

1. Bring your pace to a moderate intensity (RPE 6). Hold for 2 minutes.
2. Increase your pace to a challenging intensity (RPE 7). Hold for 2 minutes.
3. Increase your pace to a very challenging intensity (RPE 8). Hold for 2 minutes.
4. Increase your pace to an uncomfortable yet manageable intensity (RPE 9). Hold for 2 minutes.
5. Repeat ladder 2–3 times.
6. Cool down for 2–5 minutes at a comfortable pace (RPE 3–4).

Week 6

1. Bring your pace to a moderate intensity (RPE 6). Hold for 3 minutes.
2. Increase your pace to a challenging intensity (RPE 7). Hold for 3 minutes.
3. Increase your pace to a very challenging intensity (RPE 8). Hold for 3 minutes.
4. Increase your pace to an uncomfortable yet manageable intensity (RPE 9). Hold for 3 minutes.
5. Repeat ladder 2–3 times.
6. Cool down for 2–5 minutes at a comfortable pace (RPE 3–4).

Week 7

1. Bring your pace to a moderate intensity (RPE 6). Hold for 3 minutes.

2. Increase your pace to a very challenging intensity (RPE 8). Hold for 4 minutes.

3. Slightly increase your pace to a more challenging intensity (RPE 8.5). Hold for 4 minutes.

4. Increase your pace to an uncomfortable yet manageable pace (RPE 9). Hold for 4 minutes.

5. Repeat ladder 2–3 times.

6. Cool down for 2–5 minutes at a comfortable pace (RPE 3–4).

Week 8:

1. Bring your pace to a challenging intensity (RPE 7). Hold for 5 minutes.

2. Increase your pace to a very challenging intensity (RPE 8). Hold for 5 minutes.

3. Increase your pace to an uncomfortable yet manageable intensity (RPE 9). Hold for 5 minutes.

4. Repeat ladder 2–3 times.

5. Cool down for 2–5 minutes at a comfortable pace (RPE 3–4).

Yoga Stretch (See pages 86–90.)

Bonus: Weeks 5–8 Go with Your Flow!

Weeks 9–12 Workouts at a Glance

Day	Warm-Up	Workout	Stretch
Monday	Mental Preparation Cardio (5–15 min.) Dynamic Stretch Power March Shoulder Circles Arm Circles Standing Trunk Twist Hip Circles Half Squat Leg Swing	Cardio-Powervals Week 9: 1 x 6 min. at a challenging pace (RPE of 7.5). Follow with 2 min. at a comfortable pace (RPE of 5) 1 x 5 min. at a very challenging pace (RPE of 8). Follow with 2 min. at a moderate pace (RPE of 5) 1 x 4 min. at a very challenging pace (RPE of 8.5). Follow with 2 min. at a moderate pace (RPE of 5) 1 x 3 min. at a very challenging pace (RPE of 8.7). Follow with 2 min. at a moderate pace (RPE of 5) 1 x 2 min. at a very challenging pace RPE of 8.8). Follow with 2 min. at a moderate pace (RPE of 5) 1 x 1 min. at an uncomfortable yet manageable pace (RPE of 9). Follow with 2 min. at a comfortable pace (RPE of 5) Week 10: 3 x 3 min. at a very challenging pace (RPE of 8.5). Follow with 2 min. at a moderate pace (RPE of 5) 3 x 2 min. at a very challenging pace (RPE of 8.8). Follow with 2 min. at a moderate pace (RPE of 5) 3 x 1 min. at an uncomfortable yet manageable pace (RPE 9). Follow with 2 min. at a moderate pace (RPE of 5) Week 11: 5 x 5 min. at a very challenging pace (RPE of 8.8). Follow with 2 min. at a moderate pace (RPE of 5) Week 12: 6 x 6 min. at a very challenging pace (RPE 8.8). Follow with 2 min. at a moderate pace (RPE of 5) Cool down 2–5 min. at a comfortable pace (RPE of 3–4) Core Circuit 2 x 10–25 abdominal crunches 2 x 30 sec.–3 min. core hold 2 x 10–25 reps. seated trunk twist 2 x 10–25 reps. abdominal rope climb 2 x 10–25 reps. abdominal bike ride with reach	Yoga Stretch Standing Mountain Pose Standing Side Bend Downward Dog Cobra Modified Pigeon Pose Bridge Pose Happy Baby Pose Cleansing Breaths
Tuesday	Mental Preparation Cardio (5–15 min.) Dynamic Stretch Power March Shoulder Circles Arm Circles Standing Trunk Twist Hip Circles Half Squat Leg Swing	Fit Fusion Circuit 2 x 10–15 reps. step climb 2 x 10–15 reps. front-side shoulder raise superset 2 x 10–15 reps. standing trunk twist with punch 2 x 10–15 reps. triceps kick back 2 x 10–15 reps. fit ball inner thigh squat 2 x 1–2 min. jump rope or modified jump rope 2 x 1–2 min. line drill or toe tap 2 x 10–15 power push-ups Aerobic Cardio 20–30 min. at a challenging pace (RPE of 7) Cool down for 3–5 min. at a comfortable pace (3–4)	Yoga Stretch Standing Mountain Pose Standing Side Bend Downward Dog Cobra Modified Pigeon Pose Bridge Pose Happy Baby Pose Cleansing Breaths

Wednesday	Mental Preparation Cardio (5–15 min.) Dynamic Stretch Power March Shoulder Circles Arm Circles Standing Trunk Twist Hip Circles Half Squat Leg Swing	Cardio-Rhythm 3–5 min. build to a very challenging pace (RPE of 8.5) Week 9: 25 min. at a very challenging pace (RPE of 8.5) Week 10: 2 x 15 min. at a very challenging pace (RPE of 8.5). Follow each with 3 min. at a comfortable pace (RPE of 3–4) Week 11: 30 min. at a challenging pace (RPE of 8.5) Week 12: 35 min. at a challenging pace (RPE of 8.5) Cool down 2–5 min. at a comfortable pace (RPE of 3–4) Core Circuit 2 x 10–25 reps. abdominal bike ride with reach 2 x 10–25 reps. Pilates reach to scissor kick superset 2 x 10–25 reps. abdominal rope climb 2 x 10–25 reps. jackknife/fit ball exchange 2 x 30 sec.–3 min. core hold	Yoga Stretch Standing Mountain Pose Standing Side Bend Downward Dog Cobra Modified Pigeon Pose Bridge Pose Happy Baby Pose Cleansing Breaths
Thursday	Rest or Active Recovery Day		
Friday	Mental Preparation Cardio (5–15 min.) Dynamic Stretch Power March Shoulder Circles Arm Circles Standing Trunk Twist Hip Circles Half Squat Leg Swing	Cardio-Ladder Week 9: • 3 min. at a challenging pace (RPE of 7) • Increase every 3 min. from a challenging to very challenging to uncomfortable yet manageable pace (RPE of 7, 8, 9) • 2 min. at a moderate pace (RPE of 6) • Repeat ladder 2 times Week 10: • 3 min. at a challenging pace (RPE of 7) • Increase every 4 min. from a challenging to very challenging to uncomfortable yet manageable pace (RPE of 7, 8, 9) • 2 min. at a moderate pace (RPE of 6) • Repeat ladder 2 times Week 11: • 3 min. at a challenging pace (RPE of 7) • Increase every 5 min. from a challenging to very challenging to uncomfortable yet manageable pace (RPE of 7, 8, 9) • 2 min. at a moderate pace (RPE of 6) • Repeat ladder 2 times Week 12: • 3 min. at a challenging pace (RPE of 7) • Increase every 6 min. from a challenging to very challenging to uncomfortable yet manageable pace (RPE of 7, 8, 9) • 2 min. at a moderate pace (RPE of 6) • Repeat ladder 2 times Cool down 2–5 min. at a comfortable pace (RPE 3–4)	Yoga Stretch Standing Mountain Pose Standing Side Bend Downward Dog Cobra Modified Pigeon Pose Bridge Pose Happy Baby Pose Cleansing Breaths
Saturday	Go with Your Flow!		
Sunday	Rest or Active Recovery Day		

Weeks 9–12 Workout Descriptions

WORKOUT 1, WEEKS 9–12: CARDIO-POWERVALS AND CORE CIRCUIT

" *We must be willing to sacrifice what we are for who we are capable of becoming.*—Coach E

Warm-Up (See Mental Preparation, Cardio Warm-Up, and Dynamic Stretch, pages 71–75.)

Cardio-Powervals

Week 9

1. 1 x 6 minutes at a challenging pace (RPE 7.5).
   Follow Powerval with 2 minutes at a moderate pace (RPE 5).
2. 1 x 5 minutes at a very challenging pace (RPE 8).
   Follow Powerval with 2 minutes at a moderate pace (RPE 5).
3. 1 x 4 minutes at a very challenging pace (RPE 8.5).
   Follow Powerval with 2 minutes at a moderate pace (RPE 5).
4. 1 x 3 minutes at a very challenging pace (RPE 8.7).
   Follow Powerval with 2 minutes at a moderate pace (RPE 5).
5. 1 x 2 minutes at a very challenging pace (RPE 8.8).
   Follow Powerval with 2 minutes at a moderate pace (RPE 5).
6. 1 x 1 minute at an uncomfortable yet manageable pace (RPE 9).
   Follow Powerval with 2 minutes at a moderate pace (RPE 5).
7. Cool down for 2–5 minutes at a comfortable pace (RPE 5).

Week 10

1. 3 x 3 minutes at a very challenging pace (RPE 8.5).
   Follow each Powerval with 2 minutes at a moderate pace (RPE 5).
2. 3 x 2 minutes at a very challenging pace (RPE 8.8).
   Follow each Powerval with 2 minutes at a moderate pace (RPE 5).

3. 3 x 1 minute at an uncomfortable yet manageable pace (RPE 9).
   Follow each Powerval with 2 minutes at a moderate pace (RPE 5).

4. Cool down for 2–5 minutes at a comfortable pace (RPE 5).

Week 11

1. 5 x 5 minutes at a very challenging pace (RPE 8.8).
   Follow each Powerval with 2 minutes at a moderate pace (RPE 5).

2. Cool down for 2–5 minutes at a comfortable pace (RPE 5).

Week 12

1. 6 x 6 minutes at a very challenging pace (RPE 8.8).
   Follow each Powerval with 2 minutes at a moderate pace (RPE 5).

2. Cool down for 2–5 minutes at a comfortable pace (RPE 5).

Core Circuit

1–3 sets of 10–25 *Abdominal Crunches* (See description on page 94.)

1–3 sets of 30 sec.–3 min. *Core Hold* (See description on page 97.)

1–3 sets of 10–25 *Seated Trunk Twists* (See description on page 118.)

1–3 sets of 10–25 reps. *Abdominal Rope Climb* (See description on page 118.)

1–3 sets of 10–25 reps. *Abdominal Bike Ride with Reach* (See description on pages 96–97.)

Yoga Stretch (See pages 86–90.)

WORKOUT 2, WEEKS 9–12: FIT FUSION CIRCUIT

> " *Trust only movement. Life happens at the level of events,*
> *not of words. Trust movements.* —Alfred Adler*

Warm-Up (See Mental Preparation, Cardio Warm-Up, and Dynamic Stretch, pages 71–75.)

Fit Fusion Circuit

Step Climb

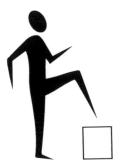

Benefits: caloric burn; strengthens and tones legs and gluteus.

Equipment: platform or step

1. Face a step or stair.
2. Step up with your right foot, followed by your left as quickly as possible as if you were running up a flight of stairs. Keep your back straight.
3. Return to the starting position by dropping your right foot followed by your left foot to the floor.
4. Repeat for 1–2 minutes. Complete 1–3 sets.

Front-Side Shoulder Raise

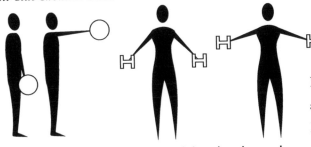

Benefits: strengthens and tones shoulders and upper back.

Equipment: free weights

1. Stand with free weights in each hand and arms by your sides.
2. Simultaneously bring up weights with both arms to the tip of your nose, keeping back straight and elbows slightly bent and locked.
3. Slowly bring arms back to your sides.

Standing Trunk Twist with Punch

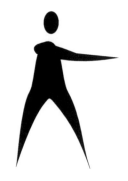

Benefits: strengthens and tones abdominals, side obliques, shoulders, and triceps.

Equipment: free weights

1. Stand with free weights by your ribs, with slight bend at your knees.
2. Keeping your lower body still, exhale and rotate at your waist while simultaneously engaging your abdominals and punching your arm forward. Hold for a 1-count. Return your arm back to your side and repeat with your other arm.
3. Repeat 10–15 times with each arm. Complete 1–3 sets.

Triceps Kick Backs

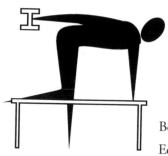

Benefits: strengthens and tones triceps.

Equipment: free weights

1. Bending at your waist, flatten your back so that it's parallel to the floor.
2. Bring your elbows up and lock them to your ribs.
3. Exhale and extend your forearms out while simultaneously turning your wrist toward the sky. Keep your upper arm still during the entire movement.
4. Hold the top of the movement for a 2-count. Inhale and slowly return to the starting position on a slow 3-count.
5. Repeat 10–15 times. Complete 1–3 sets.

Fit Ball Inner Thigh Squat (See description on page 100.)
1–3 sets of 10–15 reps.

Jump Rope (See description on page 125.)
1–3 sets of 1–2 min.

Line Drill (See description on page 123.)
1–3 sets of 1–2 min.

Power Push-Up (See description on pages 76–79.)

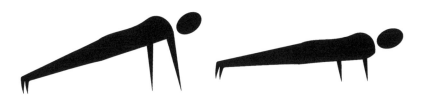

1–3 sets of 10–15 reps.

Aerobic Cardio Set
1. Choose a cardio activity.
2. Build to a challenging pace (RPE 7). Hold for 20–30 minutes.
3. Cool down for 3–5 minutes at a comfortable pace (RPE 3–4).

Yoga Stretch (See pages 86–90.)

WORKOUT 3, WEEKS 9-12: CARDIO-RHYTHM AND CORE CIRCUIT

❝ *Dreams pass into the reality of action. From the action stems the dream again; and this interdependence produces the highest form of living.* —Anaïs Nin

Warm-Up (See Mental Preparation, Cardio Warm-Up, and Dynamic Stretch, pages 71–75.)

Cardio-Rhythm
Week 9

1. Take 3–5 minutes to slowly build up to a very challenging pace (RPE 8.5).
2. Continue for 25 minutes at a very challenging pace (RPE 8.5).
3. Cool down for 2–5 minutes at a comfortable pace (RPE 3–4).

Week 10

1. Take 3–5 minutes to slowly build up to a very challenging pace (RPE 8.5).
2. Complete 2 x 15-minute intervals at a very challenging pace (RPE 8.5). Follow each interval with 3 minutes recovery at a comfortable pace (RPE 3–4).
3. Cool down for 2–5 minutes at a comfortable pace (RPE 3–4).

Week 11

1. Take 3–5 minutes to slowly build up to a very challenging pace (RPE 8.5).
2. Continue for 30 minutes at a very challenging pace (RPE 8.5).
3. Cool down for 2–5 minutes at a comfortable pace (RPE 5).

Week 12

1. Take 3–5 minutes to slowly build up to a very challenging pace (RPE 8.5).
2. Continue for 35 minutes at a very challenging pace (RPE 8.5).
3. Cool down for 2–5 minutes at a comfortable pace (RPE 3–4).

Core Circuit

1–3 sets of 10–25 reps. *Abdominal Bike Ride with Reach* (See description on pages 96–97.)

1–3 sets of 10–25 reps. *Pilates Reach to Scissor Kick Superset* (See description on page 96.)

1–3 sets of 10–25 reps. *Abdominal Rope Climb* (See description on pages 118–119.)

1–3 sets of 10–25 reps. *Jackknife/Fit Ball Exchange* (See description on pages 117–118.)

1–2 sets of 30 sec.–3 min. *Core Hold* (See description on page 97.)

Yoga Stretch (See pages 86–90.)

WORKOUT 4, WEEKS 9–12: CARDIO-LADDER

There isn't anything that isn't made easier through constant familiarity and training. Through training, we can change; we can transform ourselves. — Dalai Lama

Warm-Up (See Mental Preparation, Cardio Warm-Up, and Dynamic Stretch, pages 71–72.)

Week 9

1. Bring your RPE up to a challenging pace (RPE 7) and hold for 3 minutes.
2. Increase your RPE every 3 minutes from a challenging to very challenging to an uncomfortable yet manageable pace, following this pattern: RPE of 7, 8, 9.
3. Then decrease your intensity to a moderate pace (RPE 6) and hold for 2 minutes.
4. Repeat 1–3 times.
5. Cool down for 2–5 minutes at a comfortable pace (RPE 3–4).

Week 10

1. Bring your RPE up to a challenging pace (RPE 7) and hold for 3 minutes.
2. Increase your RPE every 4 minutes from a challenging to very challenging to an uncomfortable yet manageable pace, following this pattern: RPE of 7, 8, 9.
3. Then decrease your intensity to a moderate pace (RPE 6) and hold for 2 minutes.
4. Repeat 1–3 times.
5. Cool down for 2–5 minutes at a comfortable pace (RPE 3–4).

Week 11

1. Bring your RPE up to a challenging pace (RPE 7) and hold for 3 minutes.

2. Increase your RPE every 5 minutes from a challenging to very challenging to an uncomfortable yet manageable pace, following this pattern: RPE of 7, 8, 9.

3. Then decrease your intensity to a moderate pace (RPE 6) and hold for 2 minutes.

4. Repeat 1–3 times.

5. Cool down for 2–5 minutes at a comfortable pace (RPE 3–4).

Week 12

1. Bring your RPE up to a challenging pace (RPE 7) and hold for 3 minutes.

2. Increase your RPE every 6 minutes from a challenging to very challenging to an uncomfortable yet manageable pace, following this pattern: RPE of 7, 8, 9.

3. Then decrease your intensity to a moderate pace (RPE 6) and hold for 2 minutes.

4. Repeat 1–3 times.

5. Cool down for 2–5 minutes at a comfortable pace (RPE 3–4).

Yoga Stretch (See pages 86–90.)

Bonus: Weeks 9–12 Go with Your Flow!

Fit 'n Fifteen Express Circuits

The Fit 'n Fifteen Express is a 15-minute, 5-exercise circuit series.

Suggestions:

• Perform each exercise for 1–2 minutes or until you reach muscular failure and cannot perform another repetition.

• Complete 2 sets of each exercise with a 30-second rest between exercises.

Benefits:

• Requires no equipment and can be done anywhere. Perfect for those who are traveling or prefer to train outside or at home.

• Can be used instead of or combined with the health club workout to create your personal breakthrough fitness plan.

• Highly effective for all ages and athletic abilities.

FIT 'N FIFTEEN EXPRESS WORKOUT 1

Warm-Up (See Mental Preparation, Cardio Warm-Up, and Dynamic Stretch, pages 71–75.)

Express Circuit

Turbo Squat

With arms straight out, inhale and perform a squat. At the bottom of the movement, exhale and explode up to your starting position. Repeat rapidly. Be mindful not to allow your knees to come over your toes.

Suggestion: Take note of how many you can do in a 1-minute period and seek to beat your number of repetitions in subsequent sets.

Power Push-Ups (See description on pages 76–79.)

Earth-Sky Jumps (See description on page 123.)

Abdominal Bike Ride with Reach (See description on pages 96–97.)

Stair Climbers (See description on page 126.)

Yoga Stretch (See pages 86–90.)

FIT 'N FIFTEEN EXPRESS WORKOUT 2

Warm-Up (See Mental Preparation, Cardio Warm-Up, and Dynamic Stretch, pages 71–75.)

Express Circuit

Turbo Squat-Double Punch

1. Begin with your hands by your mid ribs.
2. Inhale and squat down.
3. On the exhale, stand up rapidly and double punch by leading with your right hand and following with your left hand.
4. Repeat rapidly.

Scissor Jumps (See description on page 124.)

Chair Pose (See description on page 102.)

Squat-Thrust-Jump (See description on pages 126–127.)

Elbow to Knee Turbo Twist

1. Begin with your feet shoulder-width apart and arms out with a 90-degree bend at your elbow.

2. Exhale and rapidly raise your left knee toward your right elbow. Inhale and return to your starting position.

3. Repeat rapidly alternating elbows and knees.

Yoga Stretch (See pages 86–90.)

FIT 'N FIFTEEN EXPRESS WORKOUT 3:

Warm-Up (See Mental Preparation, Cardio Warm-Up, and Dynamic Stretch, pages 71–75.)

Express Circuit

Step-Ups (See description on page 98.)

Jump Rope (See description on page 125.)

Boat Pose (See description on page 95.)

Triceps Dip (See description on page 80.)

Core Hold (See description on page 97.)

Yoga Stretch (See pages 86–90.)

FIT 'N FIFTEEN EXPRESS WORKOUT 4

Warm-Up (See Mental Preparation, Cardio Warm-Up, and Dynamic Stretch, pages 71–75.)

Express Circuit

Power Push-Ups (See description on pages 76–79.)

Line Drill (See description on page 123.)

Bird-Dog Pose (See description on page 113.)

Abdominal Crunches (See description on page 94.)

Fit Ball Inner Thigh Squats (See description on page 100.)

Yoga Stretch (See pages 86–90.)

FIT 'N FIFTEEN EXPRESS WORKOUT 5

Warm-Up (See Mental Preparation, Cardio Warm-Up, and Dynamic Stretch, pages 71–75.)

Express Circuit
Power Push-Ups (See description on pages 76–79.)
Foot Fire (See description on page 127.)
Inner and Outer Thigh Cross (See description on pages 124–125.)
Pilates Reach to Scissor Kick Superset (See description on page 96.)
Abdominal Bike Ride with Reach (See description on pages 96–97.)

Yoga Stretch (See pages 86–90.)

For free Coach Erik training videos and exercise demonstrations, I invite you to go to www.coacherik.com.

Fitness Journal

During your 12-week jump-start fitness program, I invite you to take a few minutes each day to track your workouts and jot down any thoughts, successes, and challenges you experience along the way.

Example:

Date: / /	Workout	Notes
Monday		

Tuesday		
Wednesday		
Thursday		
Friday		
Saturday		
Sunday		

Part III
Mindful Eating

> **Mindful eating empowers you to both enjoy food and tap into its power to nourish, heal, and energize your body and your life.** —*Coach E*

For many, the greatest obstacle in their quest to live a fit, vital, and empowered life is their relationship with food. The *Merriam-Webster Dictionary* defines nutrition as "the act or process of nourishing or being nourished; *specifically* the sum of the processes by which an animal or plant takes in and utilizes food substances." As straightforward as this sounds, when we think about what drives our food choices, the process of nourishing our bodies is often complex and multi-layered. The reason is that food often means more to us than simply nourishing our bodies and eating what we need to survive.

Food can mean:

- enjoyment
- fuel
- vitality
- ritual
- reward
- guilt

- comfort
- punishment
- control
- social/spiritual values
- beliefs about what supports or hinders our health

We all have our own personal relationship and history with food. Adding another layer to that are the conflicting messages we get from our family, "experts," friends, media, and society as a whole. On one hand, we're taught to value foods that are good for us, while on the other hand, we're surrounded by low-nutrient foods—super-sized and super-fast foods that make it difficult to maintain a healthful lifestyle.

To the rescue is the billion-dollar-a-year diet industry, offering us an abundance of information and a multitude of diets, each claiming to be the perfect way to lose weight and get fit. There's the low-fat diet, the no-fat diet, the no-carbohydrate diet, the liquid diet, the raw food diet . . . and the list goes on and on.

So what's the answer? Which diet will support your health and fitness goals, *and* allow you to enjoy food in the process? Does it even exist? Well, yes and no. There is a way to live a fit and well life without losing your love of food, but it's not a "diet" at all.

Make Your Nourishment Connection

Most diets focus primarily on controlling what you eat. Over time, this often results in deprived, guilty, and frustrated feelings. Mindful eating invites you to create a harmonious relationship with food that is void of judgment or self-criticism. It empowers you to enjoy all that food has to offer while nourishing, healing, and energizing your body and your life.

Mindful Eating can help you:

- eat in a way that supports abundant fitness and wellness.
- cultivate a positive, empowering relationship with food that does not require obsessive dieting, deprivation, or "willpower."
- make food choices from a position of strength and awareness.

Overview

This chapter is broken down into four sections:

- Section I introduces the concept of mindful eating and invites you to heal and strengthen your current relationship with food.
- Section II offers basic guidelines for nourishing your body and energizing your life.
- Section III explores the 8 superfoods.
- Section IV offers you sample meal and recipe suggestions.

For additional tips, support, community, and coaching, I invite you to visit the fit and well team website at www.coacherik.com.

Section I: An Introduction to Mindful Eating

I define mindful eating as deliberately paying attention to what's going on within you and around you during all facets of your eating experience. The cornerstone of mindful eating is awareness. For example, an awareness of hunger, fullness, cravings, mood, taste, surroundings, etc. Deliberate awareness promotes balance, choice, wisdom, and acceptance. Over time, deliberate awareness can free you of reactive habitual patterns that affect how you think, feel, and act.

As you become more attuned to the direct experience of eating and the accompanying feelings of health and vitality, you gain insight into how you can achieve specific fitness and wellness goals without dieting. This intuitive approach is internally directed and gives you the power to make choices that are void of "good" and "bad" as well as self-criticism and judgment.

Note: In some cases addictive behavior takes over and a person no longer has control over their food choices. These situations may require more focused attention. If this resonates with you, I invite you to consider two transformative eating- and support-based programs: www.overeaters.org and www.foodaddicts.org.

SUGGESTIONS FOR EATING MORE MINDFULLY

Tune In Before Eating

Pay deliberate attention to what is present for you internally before eating. I invite you to use the following questions as a guide:

- Am I hungry?
- What is my body asking for?
- What is my mood? What's going on with me right now?
- Is my mood driving my thoughts about what to eat?

CREATE A MINDFUL EATING ENVIRONMENT

Notice your environment. Are you distracted by the television or computer? Are you eating on the go? Are you present to the experience of eating right now?

I invite you to create an environment that supports mindful eating by contemplating the following question: How can I create an environment right now that is conducive to mindful eating?

HONOR YOUR FOOD

I invite you to take a moment and honor the food you're about to eat. Think about where that food comes from. Think about everything that had to happen for that food to get to your plate. One way to do this is through a simple prayer: "I am grateful for the food I am about to eat." Honoring your food is another way of honoring yourself.

TUNE IN WHILE YOU'RE EATING

Focus on sensations, tastes, smells, and feelings of fullness. I invite you to put down your utensils between bites. Chew, savor, and delight in the eating experience. Periodically check in with your stomach. Are you full?

TUNE IN AFTER YOU EAT

Without guilt or judgment I invite you to contemplate the following questions:

- How do I feel? Energized? Sluggish? Vital? Full? Hungry?
- What can I take away from this eating experience that can help me eat more mindfully in the future?

Heal and Strengthen Your Relationship with Food

This section is intended to help you eat with more joy and mindfulness by offering ways to heal and strengthen your relationship with food.

The first step is to become aware of what food represents to you. Contemplate your current relationship with food using the following questions as a guide.

Spend a comfortable amount of time getting into a state of relaxation and presence. Consider everything that comes to mind without judgment or self-criticism.

1. What does food mean to you?

_____

_____

_____

_____

2. In what ways do your feelings about food support and/or limit you?

_____

_____

_____

_____

Being conscious of your relationship with food and the choices you make is key to empowerment.

This relationship can range from simple to complex. Being aware of your choices puts you in a position of power, regardless of the choices you make. Remember mindfulness is not about being perfect, it's about being deliberately aware.

Resolve Inner Conflicts Using Your Whole Power Provisions

Willpower requires a tremendous amount of emotional energy and, in my experience, does not work long term. It assumes you're holding yourself back from something you really want. Acting from your whole power helps you make choices not because you have to, but because you want to. This happens as you consistently make mindful choices that are congruent with your intention and vision. On a deeper level, the shift occurs as you realize that making aligned choices feels better than momentary gratification. To realize this you have to have the experience of feeling good when you make an empowered choice. I suggest you anchor a feel-good empowered event by using the emotional anchoring exercise on page 39. Remember, you deserve to feel good . . . all the time! Commit to making choices that make you feel good and empowered.

Your Turn

1. Think about times when a food choice (or combination of food choices) limited you from moving toward the person you wanted to be. Were those choices coming from a place of self-care or were you managing an uncomfortable emotional state?

   _____

   _____

   _____

   _____

2. If they were coming from a place of managing emotions, what were you fearful of confronting? What was the underlying positive intent of the action? (For example: to help you get through a challenging day at work.) Name it. Feel it. Own it. What would it mean to let go of the old way of coping and to choose another more empowering way of dealing with challenging situations? What action needs to be taken here in spite of fear? What new evidence needs to be created?

   _____

   _____

_____

_____

_____

_____

3. Revisit Provision II, in particular the Break Through Limiting Habits exercises on pages 37–38. Explore how food has served you both positively and negatively. What would your intended transformed self do?

_____

_____

_____

_____

4. If you've relied on willpower in the past to abstain from certain foods, what would it mean to now rely on Self-Care in Action? Remember, SCIA is based on the question, _How can I value and care for myself in this moment in a way that keeps me in line with my intention and vision?_

_____

_____

_____

_____

_____

Put your new ways of coping into action. Notice how it feels to operate from a place of power and love.

Success Story
Sandra

My client Sandra's story is an example of how you can use a past model of success to break through current challenges. When I first met with Sandra, she had hit a fitness plateau. She wanted to transform her body and get back into running, which she had been told she would never be able to do after having back surgery in her late twenties. Armed with her empowerment provisions (Intention, Vision, Belief, SCIA, and Positive Attitude), Sandra broke through her training plateau in a major way. She not only transformed her body, but she went on to run five Boston Marathons. After she reached her goals, though, she found herself sabotaging her success with snacking and late-night binge eating. This habit undercut her success and prevented her from living the life she wanted. Sandra overcame this challenge by applying the same success tools she used in her 90-day start-up fitness program.

The first step was to get in touch with what snacking and binging meant to her. For Sandra, late-night eating meant ritual, reward, comfort, and boredom. The next step was to come up with alternative mindful choices that did not require deprivation and willpower. This meant having enjoyable foods available to her like pre-cut fruit, vegetables, and popcorn. The third step was to reconnect to her whole power by applying the principals of Intention, Vision, Belief, SCIA, and Attitude. This process helped her recall the tenacity, determination, and focus that had helped her become successful in the past and use it to take control of the habit that was sabotaging her success in the present.

Your Turn

Success leaves clues. Can you remember a time in your life when you were connected to your whole power and took inspired action toward your intention? Is there anything from that experience that can be applied to challenges you may have with mindful eating?

_____

_____

_____

_____

_____

 Perfectionism is the voice of the oppressor. —Anne Lamott

Joy of Eating

Sometimes it's not about coping at all, but simply wanting to enjoy certain foods that may not perfectly align with your intention and vision. Enjoying birthday cake or a family pizza party, for example. Thoughts of having to be "perfect" can lead to feelings of deprivation and guilt if you mindlessly decide to partake.

When you take ownership of your choices in advance, you operate from a position of mindfulness versus willpower. Feeling like you must forgo foods you enjoy can set you up for the roller coaster ride of feeling deprived, and then caving in: abstinence . . . followed by binging. *Get off the ride once and for all!* I invite you to enjoy food! Use your mindfulness techniques to find the balance that feels right to you.

Sometimes the inner conflict is around sabotaging your success. (See Fear of Success on pages 43–44.) For example, consistently eating in ways you know will consciously or subconsciously undo your hard-earned progress.

At its core, sabotaging your success is about not feeling deserving of success. Remember, to manifest your intention and vision, you must believe you deserve it. Sometimes it takes time to grow into the feeling of power and happiness that comes from consistent SCIA. Sit with it. Allow it to wash over you. Over time it will feel natural. The miracle is nothing less than a complete paradigm shift in the way you see yourself and how you relate to food. Allow yourself to be uncomfortable. Don't quit . . . the miracle is on its way!

Success Story
Ceila

Ceila had been dieting most of her adult life. For years, she was a yo-yo dieter, losing weight with various diets only to regain it. (Sound familiar?) Her breakthrough came by developing deliberate awareness, a new empowered relationship with food, and a personal weekly meal plan. While Ceila was not always "perfect" on her plan, she learned from her setbacks and over time developed a consistent balance. To date, Ceila has transformed her body and enjoys explosive energy and vitality. All because she makes conscious food choices from a position of mindfulness and personal strength as opposed to relying on willpower.

Your Turn

Now that you've created awareness around your current relationship with food, the next step is to define and nurture a new relationship that supports your intention *and* allows you to enjoy eating without judgment or guilt. Use the following questions to help you get in touch with your inner genius and transformed self.

1. What kind of relationship does my transformed self have with food?

_____

_____

_____

2. How does my transformed self cope with stress and anxiety without coping with food?

_____

_____

_____

3. What food choices does my transformed self make when stressed and anxious?

_____

_____

_____

4. What issues/relationships underlying limiting food choices has my transformed self addressed and begun to heal?

_____

_____

_____

5. How does my transformed self stay mindful? How does she/he approach the experience of eating?

_____

_____

_____

In order to stay mindful and empowered during challenging food situations (like going out to eat or a holiday party), it's important to intend rather than react. Intending means you've thought about the situation in advance and have a plan of action. Reacting means you have no plan and act according to how you feel in the moment. Can you think of a situation where you intended or reacted during a challenging food situation?

_____

_____

_____

Ideas for intending versus reacting when making food choices:

1. First thing in the morning ask yourself, How do I intend to eat today? Am I prepared to follow through on this intention?

2. Before entering a challenging food situation, ask your inner genius the following questions:

- What choices do I intend to make here?

- What can I do to stay mindful in this situation?
- What can I do in advance of this situation to prepare?

Listen to your inner genius and follow through. Feel the power of deciding how you've chosen to relate to food today. Food does not have to be the enemy. In fact, food can be your supreme ally. By cultivating a healthy relationship with food, you have the power to heal, energize, and change your mood, as well as transform your physique and your life.

If you make a choice that doesn't feel good, let it go and move on. Feeling guilty or bad does nothing to enhance the situation. What has this situation taught you? How can you use what you've learned going forward? Release yourself from guilt. Let it go and get back into your flow! A great way to do this is to continue to "work" your empowerment provisions. Perhaps a new clear decision or a commitment to a positive attitude is necessary? Maybe a new purpose charged with positive emotion is called for?

> " *Our greatest glory is not in never failing, but in rising up every time we fail.* — Ralph Waldo Emerson

Section II: Nourish Your Body and Energize Your Life: A Basic Food Guide

The Nourish Your Body and Energize Your Life Food Guide is based on the question, What nourishing food choices can I make over the next 90 days and beyond to support my health and create abundant energy and vitality in my life? While there are no one-size-fits-all answers to this question, the invitations that follow are intended to serve as a solid starting point as you develop a mindful and empowered way of eating that works for you.

Invitation 1: Eat Predominantly Whole Foods

Whole foods are foods that are in (or close to) their natural state or, as I like to say, "of the earth." Some examples include: naturally/organically grown fruits and vegetables; unprocessed poultry and fish; legumes such as beans and lentils; and whole grains such as oats and brown rice. Whole foods are unprocessed, or minimally processed, and unrefined. Typically, they contain no added sugar or salt and provide you with essential vitamins, minerals, and disease-fighting agents.

Invitation 2: Drink Up

Hydration is essential to nearly every function of the human body and is vital for survival. Here's a snapshot:

- 55–75% of your body weight is composed of water.
- Water helps cleanse your body of toxins, bring nutrients and oxygen to cells, protect major organs, lubricate joints, and regulate body temperature.
- Often when you feel hungry, your body is really asking for water.
- Chronic dehydration limits your body's ability to metabolize fat and promotes water retention. Staying hydrated supports fat metabolism, promotes fluid release, and reduces bloating. Yes, drinking more water helps you release water, lose weight, and feel less bloated!
- Adequate hydration has been linked to increased energy, increased concentration, and feelings of well-being.
- A 2% change in body weight due to dehydration can cause a 10–15% decrease in athletic performance, focus, and energy.
- Most people satisfy 15–20% of their fluid needs from the food they eat. Fruits and vegetables are composed of up to 90% water.
- The latest research suggests caffeinated beverages such as tea and coffee when consumed in moderation do not dehydrate you as once suggested and do "count" toward optimal fluid suggestions.

- Alcoholic beverages act as a diuretic and do not count toward your optimal suggested fluid intake. However, studies suggest that there may be health benefits to drinking alcohol in moderation.

Suggestions for ensuring you are drinking enough fluids:
- Fluid needs vary. However, a good starting point is 64 ounces (2 liters) of total fluid per day for women and 94 fluid ounces (3 liters) per day for men. Note: This is in addition to the fluid you drink during exercise. (See below.)
- The color of your urine is a good indicator of hydration. If your urine is pale yellow to clear, you're on track. If it's dark yellow to maple syrup color . . . drink up!
- Use thirst as an indicator of hydration. If you're feeling thirsty, chances are you're already heading toward dehydration.
- Carry water with you at all times. Don't worry, as soon as your body adjusts you won't have to urinate as frequently, as your body will begin to excrete more volume each time.
- Drink a tall glass of cold water first thing in the morning to help you rehydrate and rejuvenate.
- Drink consistently throughout the day. Drink a tall glass of water before each meal to help curb overeating.
- Drink 16–24 ounces of water 2 hours prior to exercising and then another 8–16 ounces of water 15–30 minutes before exercising.

To get a good estimate of optimal fluid intake during exercise, I also suggest doing an hourly sweat rate test:
1. Weigh yourself naked before you exercise.
2. Weigh yourself naked after you exercise for 1 hour. Subtract your weight after exercise from your weight before exercise, e.g., 143 lbs. – 142 lbs. = 1 lb.
3. Convert your weight loss into ounces, e.g., 1 lb. = 16 oz.
4. Add the amount of ounces lost to the number of ounces you drank during the hour, e.g., 16 oz. + 8 oz. = 24 oz. This is your sweat rate.
5. For optimal hydration, you want your hourly sweat rate to equal your hourly water intake.

Weight Before – Weight After	Loss in Ounces	Water Intake	Loss + Water Intake = Sweat Rate
143 lbs. – 142 lbs. = 1 lb.	1 lb. = 16 oz.	8 oz.	16 oz. + 8 oz. = 24 oz.

You *can* drink too much water. Hyponatremia (water intoxication) occurs when water intake dilutes your electrolyte balance, causing low sodium levels in your blood. This condition typically occurs during extended cardiovascular exercise sessions (over 90 minutes). Alternating between water and sports drinks with sodium to meet your optimal hourly water intake may reduce the risk of hyponatremia.

Invitation 3: Take a Multivitamin Every Day

A basic multivitamin is a great way to ensure you're getting all the nutrients you need to support your health. While a multivitamin is not a substitute for nutrients found in food, you can think of it as a nutrition insurance policy that fills in any daily nutrient gaps.

Note: If you have special concerns or are pregnant, ask your doctor about a multivitamin that's right for you.

Invitation 4: Eat Throughout the Day

Eating small mini-meals every 2–3 hours also provides you with a steady stream of energy, reducing sudden drops in blood sugar and physiological food cravings. Your body will also be able to better absorb vitamins and minerals. On the other hand, skipping meals and drastically reducing your calories puts your body into famine mode. When your body is in famine mode, it holds on to calories in the form of body fat as a survival technique.

The hardest part of "dieting" for most people is dealing with the physiological cravings: "I'm starving . . . a candy bar would do the trick!" as well as the psychological cravings: "Forget it! I'm totally stressed. Where are those chips?" Taking the physiological cravings out of the picture by committing to eat every few hours gives you more mental space to eat mindfully and make choices from a position of strength and intention.

The beauty is that you can decide to eat all day long, burn more calories, and efficiently absorb key nutrients for health and vitality. All it takes is a clear decision and some basic planning. (See Section III and IV for ideas and suggestions.)

Invitation 5: Be Mindful of Your Food Portions

Being mindful of your portions is a fantastic tool for weight management and lifelong health. A simple and effective way to measure your portions is to use the hand method. For example, a mini-meal portion of chicken may be no larger than the size of your palm. A mini-meal portion potato may be the size of your fist. A mini-meal portion of vegetables may be up to the size of your entire hand. You can find examples of the hand method and more specific ways of measuring portion sizes in Section III: 8 Superfoods.

Note: The key is to stay mindful and listen to your body's intuitive genius. If you choose to use the hand method to frame portion sizes and still feel hungry, I suggest asking yourself, *Is this my body or my mind asking for more?* If the answer is your body, aim to make a choice that nourishes you (perhaps an extra serving of vegetables or a piece of fruit) and keeps you aligned with your intention and vision.

Invitations for staying mindful of your food portions:

- Eat throughout the day. Let's face it, when you're ravenous, portion control goes out the window. Eating consistently helps keep your blood sugar from dropping and allows you to focus on your choices versus grabbing whatever is available in the moment.
- Drink a large glass of water before you eat. Often, when you think you're hungry, your body is really asking for water. Also, water will help you feel full without adding extra calories.
- Remember to be grateful. I invite you to stay grateful for the abundance of nourishment in your life. A simple inner "thank you" can help you stay connected and mindful about portions.
- Eat consciously: Take a break from your day to make mealtime special. Turn off the television and radio. Sit down. Put your fork down and savor each bite. Engage your senses by staying present to unique tastes and smells.
- Use a smaller plate. Using a salad plate versus a large dinner plate is helpful in cutting down portion sizes without feeling deprived.
- Load up on foods that contain high fiber and water, such as fruits and vegetables. This is another great way to feel satisfied without consuming extra calories.
- Cut a typical meal in half. Eat one half and save the second half for your next mini-meal. If you're out to eat and have no control of your portion size, eat half and bring the rest home. Another possibility is to ask for a box when the meal comes and put half in the box before you begin eating.

Invitation 6: Eat an Abundance of Fruits and Vegetables Each Day
Fruits and vegetables are among the healthiest and most nutrient-dense foods in existence. They contain naturally occurring vitamins and minerals as well as disease-fighting agents called photochemicals.

Benefits of eating an abundance of fruits and vegetables:
- Weight management. Fruits and vegetables are high in fiber and water content. This can

create a feeling of fullness, which can discourage the consumption of high-calorie foods. They are also typically low in calories and fat. Keep in mind, though, that eating too much of anything can also lead to weight gain.

- Fruits and vegetables are typically low in sodium, which prevents water retention.
- Fruits are high in natural sugar and low in calories that give your body a steady stream of energy and can increase feelings of well-being.
- Eating fruits and vegetables can help lower blood pressure, slow down the aging process, and reduce the risk of cardiovascular disease, diabetes, and cancers.

Invitation 8: Eat Complex Carbohydrates

Carbohydrates come in a variety of foods. Bread, potatoes, cereal, soda, milk, beans, fruits, and vegetables all contain carbohydrates. Some carbohydrates are digested more rapidly than others. Rapid digestion will cause a more rapid rise in blood sugar, hence a greater secretion of insulin. Insulin is responsible for signaling the absorption of glucose for energy storage, typically in the form of body fat. In general, unprocessed carbohydrates (e.g., whole grains, fruit, legumes, and vegetables) tend to be broken down more slowly than foods that are processed (e.g., white bread, sugary snack foods, and soda). The key is to focus on eating complex carbohydrates, which are less processed or less refined.

Grains are the seeds of a food plant such as wheat or barley that can be cultivated for food. Rice, pasta, and bread are all considered grains. A grain is considered whole when all three parts of the grain (bran, germ, endosperm) are still intact. Oatmeal, whole grain brown rice, and popcorn are examples of whole grains.

Both whole grains and refined grains (such as white bread, white rice, and white pasta) contain carbohydrates. The difference is that refined grains lose many of their key nutrients during processing. Also, refined grains can cause a rapid spike in blood glucose, which can lead to weight gain over time. Conversely, whole grains have less of an impact on blood glucose, giving you a steady stream of energy as well as an abundance of vital nutrients and possible weight management benefits.

Benefits of whole grains:
- high in fiber, which helps you feel full
- aid in digestion and may increase metabolism
- high in disease-fighting agents, phytoestrogens, and antioxidants, which may help reduce the risk of cancers, heart disease, and diabetes
- enhance energy and strength, and may increase endurance

Invitation 9: Eat "Healthy" Fats

Fat is a vital component of a healthy diet. However, some fats are healthier than others. There are four main types of fat: polyunsaturated, monounsaturated, saturated, and trans fat.

Foods high in monounsaturated fat (found in vegetable oils, nuts, seeds, and some plant foods like avocados) and polyunsaturated fat (found in vegetable oils, fish, and other seafood) are healthy fats that provide numerous benefits:

- help lower overall cholesterol, decreasing your risk of heart disease
- help maintain optimum core body temperature
- help build cell membranes and create certain hormones
- protect organs against impact
- serve as stored energy when the body is in need
- provide a sustained energy source during endurance activities
- help absorb important vitamins such as A, B, and K, which are important for vision, bone formation, blood clotting, and nerve development
- digest slower, which can help you feel fuller longer

Foods high in saturated fat are found in most red meat, whole milk, whole cheese, and many candy bars. Saturated fat can also provide many of the same health benefits of unsaturated fat. However, when eaten in excess, saturated fats may:

- increase risk of heart disease and certain cancers
- contribute to weight gain (as can unsaturated fat when eaten in excess)

Trans fats are often found in partially hydrogenated oils, which increase a product's shelf life and reduce the need for refrigeration. Trans fats are found in foods such as potato chips, commercial baked goods, crackers, and snack foods. The good news is that more and more brands are now being produced without trans fats. If the food label says partially hydrogenated oil, then it has trans fat. I suggest staying clear of these foods. Trans fats can also raise LDL (bad cholesterol) and lower HDL (good cholesterol), which is a major risk factor associated with heart disease and stroke.

Invitation 10: Eat a Variety of Complete Proteins

Protein is considered the basic building block of the human body. Made up of amino acids, protein helps build muscle, hair, skin, blood, and internal organs. Some studies suggest that a protein-rich diet can also help curb hunger.

There are twenty amino acids required for cell growth. The body makes all but eight. The eight that are not supplied are called essential amino acids. Foods that contain essential amino acids are called complete proteins. Typically, complete proteins are found in animal products such as milk, eggs, fish, and meat. Soybeans are the only plant protein considered to be a complete protein. Complete proteins can also be formed when certain incomplete proteins are combined during the course of a day; this is helpful if you follow a vegetarian or vegan lifestyle. Below are a few suggestions:

- Combine grains and legumes: beans and brown rice; peanut butter on whole wheat bread.
- Combine seeds/nuts and legumes: peanut and sunflower trail mix or hummus on whole wheat pita bread.

Note: You may also combine small amounts of animal protein to create a complete protein. For example:

- salad with beans and a hard-boiled egg
- yogurt with granola
- oatmeal with non-fat milk
- bean-and-cheese burrito

(See *Superfoods 7 and 8* on pages 173–175 for more examples.)

Section III: The 8 Superfoods

Superfood 1: Fruit

Frequently Asked Questions

Q: Many of the popular diets out there suggest that the sugar in fruit will make it difficult to lose weight. Is this true?

A: Not if you're mindful of your portion sizes and overall caloric intake. The benefits of eating fruit far outweigh the limitations. While fruit contains natural sugar, it has less of an impact on insulin and blood glucose than refined sugar; consistent spikes in blood sugar can lead to weight gain and other health issues. In addition, eating a variety of fruits each day can have a tremendous effect on your overall health while supporting weight management.

Q: What are the best fruits for health and weight management?

A: There are benefits to eating almost every fruit. I suggest you go for variety and what's in season in your area. Some of the best options include berries, apples, watermelons, grapefruits, oranges, kiwis, and cantaloupes.

Q: How many servings of fruit should I eat each day?

A: Aim for three to four servings of fruit per day. One serving equals:

- a medium-size whole fruit, such as an apple, banana, pear, or grapefruit
- one handful of blueberries, strawberries, or grapes
- a small glass of 100% (unsweetened) fruit juice

Strategies for eating more fruit:

- Keep a bowl of fruit on the kitchen table.
- Refrigerate pre-cut fruit, ready for a snack at a moment's notice.
- Top off cereal, oatmeal, and yogurt with berries.
- Bring fruit to work to eat as a snack.
- Start your day with a fruit smoothie. (See recipe on page 178.)

Superfood 2: Vegetables

Frequently Asked Questions

Q: Which vegetables do you recommend?

A: Like fruit, nearly all vegetables have an abundance of nutritional value. Cruciferous vegetables such as broccoli, cauliflower, Brussels sprouts, kale, and bok choy have it all—vitamins, fiber, and a host of disease-fighting agents. Other powerhouse vegetables include, but are not limited to, dark green, leafy vegetables such as romaine lettuce, spinach, collard greens, mushrooms, green beans, cucumbers, tomatoes (which are technically fruit but often thought of as vegetables), yellow squash, cabbage, sprouts, and avocados. I suggest you go for variety. Think multicolor to capture all the health benefits and delicious flavors. Eat your vegetables raw or lightly steamed, as they keep more of their nutrient content than fried or over-cooked vegetables. For more ideas and the health benefits associated with different fruits and vegetables check out http://www.fruitsandveggiesmatter.gov/benefits/nutrient_guide.html.

Note: To limit the amount of pesticides and herbicides you ingest, thoroughly wash your fruits and vegetables and buy organic when possible. Some of the best fruits and vegetables to consider buying organic include: berries, peaches, apples, grapes, pears, spinach, peppers, green beans, celery, and lettuce.

Q: What about potatoes?

A: Potatoes are starchy vegetables that have gotten a bad rap with the low-carb diet craze of late. The truth is white potatoes do have a significant impact on blood glucose levels. However, they are also full of nutrients, provide sustained energy, are relatively low in calories, and have almost no fat. They are also high in fiber and protein. Two fantastic alternatives to white potatoes are sweet potatoes and yams. Both capture the benefits of a white potato but with less impact on your blood sugar level.

Q: How many servings of vegetables should I eat each day?

A: I suggest you aim for three to five servings of vegetables per day. One serving equals:
- one handful of cooked or raw vegetables
- one handful of raw salad greens
- a small glass of 100% vegetable juice
- a fist-size sweet potato or yam

Strategies for eating more vegetables:
- Add vegetables to pasta sauce or omelets.
- Make a large pot of stew or soup with seasonal vegetables.
- Add vegetables to your sandwich.
- Have cut vegetables ready and serve with your favorite low-fat bean dip.

- Cut cauliflower, broccoli, or other favorite veggies into snack pieces and bring them to work.
- Have a large salad for lunch, adding lots of veggies in addition to lettuce.

Note: For many people, it's hard getting in the recommended servings of fruits and vegetables each day. If you fall into this category, begin by integrating a total of five servings of fruits and vegetables each day. This will provide you with a huge energy boost while infusing your body with essential vitamins and minerals.

Superfood 3: Whole Grains

Frequently Asked Questions:

Q: How do you feel about low-carb diets?

A: In my opinion, it is more important to focus on the kinds of carbs you are eating as opposed to limiting your carb intake. The popularity of high-protein diets has created a "carbohydrates are bad" mentality among many Americans. The truth is that simple, refined grains such as white bread, white rice, and other simple carbs found in pastries, candy bars, and soda do indeed work against you in terms of your health and weight management. However, other types of carbohydrates such as fruits, vegetables, and whole grains promote health and vitality.

Q: How do I know whether food is whole grain and unrefined?

A: Look at the back of the food package. The first ingredient should say whole wheat or whole grain. Some food items have a combination of whole and refined grains. If there is a large whole grain stamp on the package, then the food item has at least a half serving (8 grams) or more of whole grain. Be aware that multigrain and wheat bread are not whole grains. In fact, most brown wheat bread is simply white bread that has been dyed brown!

Q: Which whole grain foods do you suggest, and how many servings should I aim for each day?

A: I suggest you aim for four to five servings of whole grains per day. One serving equals:
- one handful of brown or wild rice
- one handful of stee-cut oats (uncooked)
- one slice of whole wheat, whole rye, millet, or brown rice bread
- one handful of pasta
- one handful of quinoa (pronounced keen-wah), amaranth, barley, millet, buckwheat, bran, or bulgur
- one large handful of plain popcorn (without butter)

Strategies for eating more whole grains:

- Cook a large batch of brown rice to have ready at a moment's notice.
- Think of your whole grain and vegetable as your main dish and place them in the center of your plate.
- Have a supply of 100% whole wheat, rye, or millet bread available. Another nice option is using a whole grain tortilla (sprouted wheat or rice) instead of bread—it's a great way to make a nutritious and tasty wrap for lunch or dinner!

Superfood 4: Beans and Other Legumes

Beans, including soybeans, peas, lentils, and peanuts, are from a family of vegetables called legumes. There are numerous benefits to including legumes in your Vital Eating Plan:

- They are high in photochemicals and antioxidants, which may reduce the risk of chronic diseases such as heart disease, cancer, and obesity.
- They are low in calories, fat (with the exception of peanuts, which are high in "healthy fats"), and sodium. They also contain no cholesterol and are high in fiber, making them a fantastic weight management food.
- They are complex carbohydrates. Complex carbohydrates provide a slow release of energy without spiking insulin levels that often send the calorie-storing signal to the body.
- They are high in protein, making them a quality alternative to meat when combined with another incomplete, nutrient-rich protein such as brown rice.

Strategies for eating more legumes:

- Prepare soups and other dishes that feature legumes.
- Add chickpeas or black beans to salads.
- Snack on homemade nut mix instead of pretzels or chips.

Frequently Asked Questions:

Q: Which legumes do you recommend and how many servings should I eat each week?

A: Aim for four to six servings of legumes per week. One serving equals:

- a small handful of cooked or canned black beans, soybeans/edamame, garbanzo beans (chickpeas), lima beans, black-eyed peas, kidney beans, pinto beans, adzuki beans, or mung beans
- a large handful of split, yellow, green peas, or snap peas
- a handful of red, brown, or green lentils

- 1 tsp. peanut butter
- 7–10 unsalted raw peanuts

Superfood 5: Healthy Oils

Many of the healthiest cooking oils are derived from plants. Here are some of my favorites:

Olive oil is a plant-based oil that is rich in monounsaturated fats and phytochemicals (cancer and inflammation fighting agents); it also adds taste and texture to your food.

Flaxseed oil is also a plant-based oil that is rich in essential omega-3 and omega-6 fatty acids. These acids are not made by the body and are required for the optimum health of nearly all body systems. Many studies also suggest that omega-3s help protect us from diseases, including cancer, heart disease, depression, and arthritis. Flaxseed oil is best consumed raw and should not be used as cooking oil.

There are three types of omega-3s: alpha-linolenic acid (ALA), which is found in flaxseed oil, walnuts, some green vegetables such as Brussels sprouts, kale, spinach, and salad greens; eicosapentaenoic acid (EPA); and docosahexaenoic acid (DHA). The latter two acids can be found in canola oil, walnuts, and oily fish such as salmon.

Sesame oil is a plant-based oil derived from sesame seeds. It is known for its healing powers and has been used for thousands of years. Sesame oil is rich in monounsaturated and polyunsaturated fats, is a potent antioxidant, and is a good source of calcium. This oil also promotes healthy skin and cell rejuvenation.

Sunflower oil is a plant-based oil derived from sunflower seeds. It is low in saturated fats and high in polyunsaturated fats; it is also known for its clean, light taste. This oil may help lower cholesterol and, in turn, lower your risk of heart disease.

Superfood 6: Nuts and Seeds

Nuts and seeds are high in calories and fats, yet both pack a healthy punch when eaten in moderation.

Nuts and seeds are:

- loaded with polyunsaturated and monounsaturated fats
- one of the best sources of protein from plants
- rich in fiber and disease-fighting antioxidants
- known to help lower LDL (unhealthy cholesterol) and decrease the risk of heart disease

Some of the healthiest nuts and seeds include: almonds, cashews, hazelnuts, peanuts, walnuts, flax seeds, pumpkin seeds, pistachios, and sunflower seeds.

Suggestions for eating more healthy nuts or seeds:

- Look for whole, multigrain breads made with nuts or seeds.
- Eat raw nuts or seeds as a quick and filling snack.
- Top off oatmeal, whole-grain pancakes, steamed vegetables, salads, or other dishes with nuts or seeds.

Frequently Asked Question

Q: How many servings of healthy oils, nuts, and seeds should I aim for per week?

A: Aim for two to four total combined servings of oils, nuts, and seeds per week. One serving equals:

- one teaspoon of olive or sunflower oil
- one teaspoon of flax seed oil
- a very small handful of nuts or seeds (or 7–10)
- 1 tsp. of unsweetened, raw almond butter

Superfood 7: Fish, Eggs, and Lean Meats

Fish, eggs, and other lean meats, such as poultry, are typically low in saturated fat and provide a high-quality, complete protein.

Suggestions for incorporating fish, eggs, and lean meats into your diet:

- For chicken and turkey, choose white meat without the skin, which is typically loaded with saturated fat. Also consider buying organically-raised meat, as most animals from commercial farms are treated with antibiotics and hormones, which studies suggest may have adverse health effects.
- Oily fish such as salmon, lake trout, eel, herring, and anchovies are excellent sources of protein and polyunsaturated fats. Many fish today, however, carry harmful metals such as mercury. Choose fish that are typically low in heavy metals like the oily fish listed above as well as cod, flounder, canned light tuna, halibut, haddock, and shellfish. Also, buy wild fish whenever possible. Fish that comes from aquaculture farms usually contain antibiotics used to stave off infection, which can be detrimental to humans. The American Heart Association suggests eating fatty fish at least two times per week.

Note: If you are pregnant or could become pregnant, consult your doctor about specific seafood recommendations. For further information about the safety of locally caught fish and shellfish, visit the Environmental Protection Agency's Fish Advisory website (www.epa.gov/ost/fish) or contact your state or local health department.

- Limit red meat and avoid processed meat, such as hot dogs, bacon, and deli meat, which has been linked to increasing the risk of cancer and heart disease. Some of the leanest red meat options include pork tenderloin, extra lean ground beef, and eye of round cut steak. Whenever possible, buy grass-fed meat because the animal's diet directly impacts its nutritional content. For more check out www.eatwild.com/basics.html.
- Use egg yolks sparingly as they have a high concentration of cholesterol. Instead, eat only egg whites or combine two egg whites with one whole egg when cooking or baking. Whenever possible, buy natural, free-range eggs.
- Soy-based products such as tofu and soy milk are complete protein alternatives to meat and dairy. However, there is controversy surrounding the effects of soy and soy-based products on the body. Many studies suggest that soy should be eaten in moderation (two to four servings per week).

Frequently Asked Question

Q: How many servings of fish, eggs, and lean meat should I eat per week?

A: Aim for two to three servings of fish, three to four eggs, and two to three servings of lean meat per week. One serving equals a palm-sized portion of the following:

- round steak
- 96% lean ground beef
- lean ground turkey
- lean fish (e.g., cod, flounder, and sea bass)
- oily fish (e.g., salmon)
- turkey breast
- skinless chicken breast
- tofu or tempeh

Superfood 8: Low- and Non-Fat Dairy

Low- and non-fat dairy products, such as yogurt, milk, and cheese offer high-quality complete protein with a host of possible health benefits:

- Some studies suggest that the active live cultures (good bacteria) found in yogurt can help combat gastrointestinal disorders, prevent infections, and boost your immune system.
- Low- or non-fat dairy products are high in calcium, which may help prevent osteoporosis.
- Low- and non-fat dairy may reduce the risk of high blood pressure.

Suggestions for eating low- and non-fat dairy:

- Look for "live active cultures" or "probiotics" on yogurt containers.
- Choose organic when possible. Cows that yield organic dairy eat pesticide-free grass and are not given synthetic hormones and antibiotics.
- Two solid milk alternatives include almond or rice milk. I suggest looking for brands that are fortified with calcium as some brands have no calcium at all.

Frequently Asked Question

Q: How many servings of dairy should I aim for each week?

A: Aim for three to four servings per week.

One serving equals:

- one cup milk or yogurt
- one thumb-size cube of low-fat cheese

For more information on specific recommended serving sizes, take a look at http://www.mypyramid.gov.

Section IV: Sample Meal and Recipe Suggestions

The key to developing a new way of eating for life is to stay open and flexible. There is no "right way," only a way that is right for you. I suggest you take the fundamentals and work them into your life in a way that resonates with you. Allow *your* way to emerge. Some people find it helpful to keep a food log while others are successful by keeping things more fluid. Stay present. Notice what is and is not working, and be flexible enough to change your approach when you feel it's necessary.

Suggestions for starting your Vital Eating Plan:

- Develop a meal plan at the beginning of each week that supports your intention. Create a menu. Perhaps post it next to the refrigerator.
- Prepare foods ahead of time.
- Buy a mini cooler and bring your meals to work.
- Commit to your plan.
- Be aware of how much you are eating out. It can be challenging to manage portions while eating at restaurants.
- Document food choices in your Vital Eating Journal. Notice what is and is not working. Note your challenges and feelings around food without judgment.
  Stay flexible in your approach and learn from setbacks.

Meal Suggestions

MINI-MEAL #1

1. Egg whites on dry whole-wheat toast.
2. Egg white omelet with vegetables.
3. Breakfast burrito. (See recipe on page 178.)
4. Buckwheat pancakes with egg whites and strawberries. (See recipe on pages 178–179.)
5. Steel-cut or instant oatmeal with flaxseed, blueberries, and almonds.
6. Fruit smoothie. (See recipe on page 178.)
7. Yogurt with berries.

Note: Before eating breakfast, drink 8–12 ounces of cold water with a slice of lemon and a multivitamin.

MINI-MEAL #2

1. Piece of whole fruit.

2. Toast with almond butter.

3. Homemade trail mix with nuts, seeds, raisins, cranberries, goji berries, dried fruit, etc.

4. Hummus and raw vegetables.

5. Apple and peanut butter.

6. Non-fat cottage cheese with flaxseed and berries.

MINI-MEAL #3

1. Large salad with chicken, turkey, hard-boiled egg whites, or chunk light tuna.

2. Baked sweet potato with low-fat yogurt.

3. Hummus or tuna roll-up with salad greens, tomato, cucumber, and low-fat cheese.

4. Vegetable soup with chicken or tofu. (See recipe on pages 179–180.)

5. Sliced turkey sandwich with romaine lettuce or baby spinach, tomato, avocado, and sprouts.

6. Bean burrito. (See recipe on pages 180–181.)

MINI-MEAL #4

1. Fruit smoothie.

2. Vital Eating Bar. (See recipe on pages 181–182.)

3. Almond and walnut mix.

4. Baby carrots with hummus.

5. Lentil soup with a whole-wheat roll.

MINI-MEAL #5

1. Turkey burger on a whole-wheat bun with green salad or steamed vegetables.

2. Vegetarian black bean soup. (See recipe on page 180.)

3. Grilled or baked fish with cooked spinach and brown rice.

4. Green salad with cottage cheese.

5. Whole wheat pasta with lean ground turkey, beef, or tofu and vegetables.

6. Quinoa and black bean salad. (See recipe on page 182.)

7. Turkey and/or bean chili and a fresh green salad. (See recipe on pages 182–183.)

Coach E's Simple Recipes

FRUIT SMOOTHIE

Ingredients:

1 cup fruit, fresh or frozen (e.g., strawberries, blueberries, banana, pineapple, mango)

¼ cup thickener (e.g., non-fat yogurt, frozen fruit, cup of ice)

¼ cup liquid (e.g., water, juice, skim milk, rice milk)

Combine ingredients in a blender. Makes a little more than 1 glass.

Coach E's Favorite Smoothie: 1 cup orange juice, 1 cup water, ¼ cup strawberries, ¼ cup banana, and 2 ice cubes

BREAKFAST BURRITO (Makes 1 burrito.)

Ingredients:

½ cup chopped tomato

½ cup onion

3 egg whites

6-inch whole-wheat soft tortilla

½ cup non-fat cheese

2 tablespoons salsa

olive oil cooking spray

Preparation:

1. Spray olive oil to cover the bottom of a small skillet.
2. Sauté tomatoes and onion for 2–3 minutes.
3. Add in egg whites and cook for another 3 minutes.
4. Lightly toast tortilla.
5. Add egg and vegetable omelet, cheese, and salsa to middle of tortilla.
6. Fold and close.

BUCKWHEAT PANCAKES WITH EGG WHITES AND STRAWBERRIES
(Makes about 6 pancakes.)

Ingredients:

2 egg whites

1 tablespoon olive oil

½ cup non-fat milk

1 cup buckwheat flour

1 tablespoon baking soda

½ cup water

3 cups diced strawberries

Preparation:

1. In a small bowl, whisk egg whites, oil, and milk.
2. In another bowl, combine flour and baking soda.
3. Add egg white mixture to flour and stir until moistened.
4. Place a non-stick pan or griddle on medium heat.
5. Spoon ½ cup pancake batter on pan.
6. Cook until top of pancake bubbles (about 2 minutes).
7. Flip and cook the other side until bottom is browned.
8. Top with diced strawberries.

VEGETABLE SOUP WITH CHICKEN OR TOFU (Makes 12 servings.)

Ingredients:

3 medium potatoes

1 head cauliflower

2 large carrots

1 cup butternut squash

2 large celery sticks

1 large turnip

1 ½ cups rutabaga

1 chicken thigh on bone

1 tablespoon chicken broth powder

salt and pepper to taste

Preparation:

1. Chop all vegetables.
2. Cut chicken into small, bite-size pieces.
3. Place everything into a large pot and cover with water.

4. Add salt and pepper.

5. Bring soup to a boil and then simmer for 1 ½ hours.

VEGETARIAN BLACK BEAN SOUP (Makes 12 servings.)

Ingredients:

2 cups black beans

2 tablespoons olive oil

2 cups chopped red bell peppers

5 garlic cloves, minced

2 cups chopped carrots

¼ cup chopped celery

10 cups water

2 cups diced tomatoes

3 bay leaves

1 teaspoon dried cilantro

1 teaspoon dried oregano

¼ teaspoon cumin

½ teaspoon salt

½ teaspoon pepper

Preparation:

1. In a large pot, heat the beans and oil.

2. Add red peppers, garlic, carrots, onion, and celery.

3. Cover and cook for 10 minutes or until vegetables soften.

4. Add water, tomato, bay leaves, oregano, cilantro, salt, and pepper.

5. Bring soup to a boil.

6. Reduce heat and simmer for 2 hours or until beans become tender.

7. Discard bay leaves and serve.

SUPER BEAN BURRITO (Makes 4 small burritos.)

Ingredients:

2 cups cooked black or pinto beans

2 cups cooked chicken, tofu, or beef

2 cups chopped vegetables

1 cup shredded low-fat cheese (optional)

½ teaspoon cumin

½ teaspoon salt

½ teaspoon pepper

4 6-inch whole-wheat tortillas

olive oil cooking spray

toothpicks

Preparation:

1. Preheat oven to 375 degrees.
2. Spray large cookie sheet with olive oil spray.
3. In a large bowl, combine beans, meat/tofu, vegetables, cheese, and spices.
4. Divide evenly among the tortillas. Fold and hold together with toothpicks.
5. Place tortillas on the sheet and spray with olive oil.
6. Bake for 6 minutes. Turn over and bake for another 6–8 minutes.
7. Remove toothpicks and serve.

VITAL EATING BAR (Makes 12 Vital Eating Bars.)

Ingredients:

2 large bananas, mashed

½ cup unsweetened peanut butter

½ cup honey

1 teaspoon vanilla

1 cup rolled oats

½ cup whole-wheat flour

¼ cup non-fat dry milk powder

1 teaspoon ground cinnamon

¼ teaspoon baking soda

1 cup dried cranberries, raisins, or blueberries

Preparation:

1. Preheat oven to 350 degrees. Coat 2 cookie sheets with nonstick olive oil spray and set aside.
2. In a large bowl, stir together bananas, peanut butter, honey, and vanilla. In a small bowl, combine oats, flour, milk powder, cinnamon, and baking soda.

3. Stir oat mixture with banana mixture until combined. Stir in dried cranberries.
4. Using a ¼-cup measuring cup, scoop the dough and place 3 inches apart on baking sheet. Dip a spatula in water and use to flatten dough so that each is 2 inches around and 1 inch thick.
5. Bake for 14–16 minutes or until brown.

QUINOA AND BLACK BEAN SALAD (Makes 8 cups.)

Ingredients:

3 cups water

1 ½ cups quinoa

2 teaspoons salt

¼ cup olive oil

¼ cup red wine vinegar

juice from 3 limes (about 5 tbsp.)

1 ¼ tablespoons ground cumin

2 ½ cups canned black beans, rinsed and drained

1 ½ cups frozen corn

1 red bell pepper, chopped

½ red onion, chopped

2 jalapeno peppers

2 cups cilantro, chopped

Preparation:
1. In a medium saucepan, bring water to a boil.
2. Rinse quinoa under cold running water and add to saucepan with salt.
3. Cover and reduce heat to medium.
4. Cook until liquid is absorbed (about 15 minutes).
5. Combine quinoa and other ingredients in a large bowl. Let stand for 30 minutes.

TURKEY AND/OR BEAN CHILI (Makes about 12 cups.)

Ingredients:

2 large onions, chopped

1 green pepper, chopped

¼ cup olive oil

4 garlic cloves, finely chopped

1 tablespoon ground cumin

1 tablespoon dried hot red pepper flakes

2 cans crushed tomatoes

2 tablespoons tomato paste

2 cans kidney beans and/or 3–4 cups cooked low-fat, ground turkey meat

¾ cups chicken or turkey stock

2 tablespoons chili powder (up to 4 tablespoons if you like it hot)

1 tablespoon dried oregano

1 tablespoon salt

½ teaspoon black pepper

Preparation:

1. In a large pot, heat oil and add onions and green peppers. Cook over medium heat for about 5 minutes.

2. Add garlic, chili powder, cumin, and red pepper flakes. Add more olive oil if needed.

3. Add tomatoes, tomato paste, stock, beans, oregano, salt, pepper, and cooked turkey meat (optional). Reduce heat and simmer for 1 hour.

For more healthy and delicious recipe suggestions, nutrition information, and guidelines, I invite you to join us at www.coacherik.com.

Other fantastic resources include:

Books
Moran, Victoria. *The Love-Powered Diet*. New York: Lantern Books, 2000.
Richter, Henry. *Dr. Richter's Fresh Produce Guide*. Apopka, FL: Try-Foods International, Inc., 2005.
Rinzler, Carol Ann. *Nutrition for Dummies*. Hoboken, NJ: Wiley Publishing Inc., 2005.
Willet, Walter C. *Eat, Drink, and Be Healthy*. New York: Simon & Schuster, 2005.
Online
American Dietetic Association: www.eatright.org
U.S. Department of Agriculture: www.mypyramid.gov
Harvard School of Public Health Nutrition Source: www.hsph.harvard.edu/nutritionsource
Eat Wild: www.eatwild.com
Martha McKittrick, RD, CDN, CDE: www.martha-nutritionist.com

Nutrition Journal

During your 12-week jumpstart program, I invite you to take a few minutes each day to write down what you've eaten and any thoughts, successes, and challenges you experience along the way.

Example:

Date: / /	What I Ate Today	Notes
Monday	Mini-Meal 1: Mini-Meal 2: Mini-Meal 3: Mini-Meal 4: Mini Meal 5: How much water I drank today (estimated fluid ounces):	_____ _____ _____ _____ _____ _____ _____ _____ _____ _____ _____ _____ _____ _____ _____ _____

Date: / /	What I Ate Today	Notes
Tuesday	Mini-Meal 1:	_____
		_____
	Mini-Meal 2:	_____
		_____
	Mini-Meal 3:	_____
		_____
	Mini-Meal 4:	_____
		_____
	Mini-Meal 5:	_____
		_____
	How much water I drank today (estimated fluid ounces):	

Date: / /	What I Ate Today	Notes
Wednesday	Mini-Meal 1:	_____
		_____
	Mini-Meal 2:	_____
		_____
	Mini-Meal 3:	_____
		_____
	Mini-Meal 4:	_____
		_____
	Mini-Meal 5:	_____
		_____
	How much water I drank today (estimated fluid ounces):	

Date: / /	What I Ate Today	Notes
Thursday	Mini-Meal 1:	_____
		_____
	Mini-Meal 2:	_____
		_____
	Mini-Meal 3:	_____
		_____
	Mini-Meal 4:	_____
		_____
	Mini-Meal 5:	_____
		_____
	How much water I drank today (estimated fluid ounces):	

Date: / /	What I Ate Today	Notes
Friday	Mini-Meal 1:	_____
		_____
	Mini-Meal 2:	_____
		_____
	Mini-Meal 3:	_____
		_____
	Mini-Meal 4:	_____
		_____
	Mini-Meal 5:	_____
		_____
	How much water I drank today (estimated fluid ounces):	

Date: / /	What I Ate Today	Notes
Saturday	Mini-Meal 1:	
	Mini-Meal 2:	
	Mini-Meal 3:	
	Mini-Meal 4:	
	Mini-Meal 5:	
	How much water I drank today (estimated fluid ounces):	
Date: / /	What I Ate Today	Notes
Sunday	Mini-Meal 1:	
	Mini-Meal 2:	
	Mini-Meal 3:	
	Mini-Meal 4:	
	Mini-Meal 5:	
	How much water I drank today (estimated fluid ounces):	

Part IV

Living Wellness

> " *The concept of total wellness recognizes that our every thought, word, and behavior affects our greater health and well-being. And we, in turn, are affected not only emotionally but also physically and spiritually.* —Greg Anderson

Lasting transformation is a result of more than diet and exercise modifications. Your whole life needs to be nurtured. Your thoughts, relationships, sleeping patterns, work environment, and responsibilities have an immediate impact on your health and your ability to take consistent, inspired action to pursue life to its fullest potential.

The final step in making your lasting connection is what I call "living wellness." To me living wellness is the process of making active choices toward a happier, healthier, and more vital life experience. It's judgment-free Self-Care in Action (SCIA) applied to your whole life. Living wellness invites the questions, *How good can my life get? And what small, daily steps can I take to make it happen?*

The following suggestions are intended to assist you in awakening your own personal "living wellness compass." I invite you to apply these tools to areas of your life that need a boost. Keep in mind that small, consistent steps over time lead to enormous breakthroughs!

Success Story
Bill

Bill, a Type-A executive, came to me wanting to lose weight and get fit. The challenge was his life was out of balance. As a result, he was having a difficult time making choices that supported his intention and vision. When we began to look at Bill's wellness from a whole-person perspective, he could see how sleep deprivation, toxic relationships, work stress, and lack of personal time were limiting his health and overall well-being. Bill's breakthrough was the result of adopting a wellness plan. In addition to a comprehensive fitness and nutrition program, Bill's plan included strategies for managing stress, getting more sleep, healing and letting go of negative relationships, and carving out time to pursue his hobbies. In Bill's words, "The 'aha' moment for me was when

I realized I was more than just a body but an integrated whole person. By making the choice to 'live well' in all areas of my life, I could not only reach a new level of health and fitness but take my entire life to new and exciting places."

Your Turn

1. What does living wellness mean to you?

    _____

    _____

    _____

2. Why is living well essential to bringing your intention and vision to life?

    _____

    _____

    _____

3. How will living well enrich the quality of your life?

    _____

    _____

    _____

Use the following feeling scale to rate various aspects of your current wellness. The numbers are intended to represent the amount of fulfillment you feel in each area of your life.

Number	Feeling
10	I feel very connected and very fulfilled in this area of my wellness. I take personal ownership and make consistent choices to enhance this area of my well-being.
9	
8	
7	
6	
5	I feel moderately connected and fulfilled in this area of my wellness. I take inconsistent ownership and action toward enhancing this area of my well-being.
4	

3	
2	
1	I feel disconnected and unfulfilled in this area of my wellness. I don't take much ownership and action toward enhancing this area of my well-being.

How would you rate your wellness in the following areas of your life?

Social
My relationship with my partner, friends, family, community _____

Intellectual
My personal development, growth, learning _____

Spiritual
My connection to something larger than myself (i.e. spirituality, nature, causes) _____

Physical
My physical health, fitness, nutrition _____

Emotional
My attitude and habitual thoughts and feelings _____

Occupational
My career _____

Wellness Wheel

The six-dimensional wellness wheel model was created in 1976 by wellness pioneer Bill Hettler. The wheel is a great way to create a visual understanding of your current level of fulfillment in specific areas of your life. I invite you to customize the wellness wheel below by drawing a line through the number that corresponds to your ratings.

For example, my client Lisa gave herself the following ratings: social (6), intellectual (8), spiritual (4), physical (5), emotional (5), and occupational (9). Her wheel looked like this:

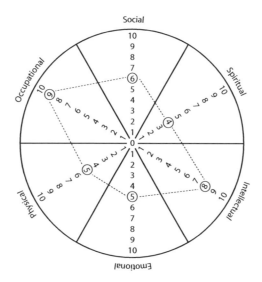

The wellness wheel helped Lisa identify areas that needed more loving attention. Her wellness plan included making time to reconnect with friends and loved ones, volunteering in a big sister program, beginning a comprehensive fitness and nutrition plan, and doing ten minutes of basic meditation each day. This whole-health approach has helped Lisa create balance and lead a more happy and fulfilled life.

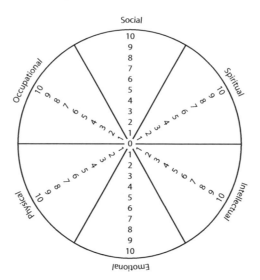

Your Turn

Using your wellness wheel as a guide, contemplate the following questions without judgment:

1. Would your current wheel create a smooth or bumpy ride through life? Is the ride currently fulfilling?

    _____

    _____

2. What needs SCIA for you to create a smoother, happier, and more fulfilled ride?

_____

_____

3. Do you feel as if you're surviving or thriving in each wellness area?

_____

_____

4. Are you ready, almost ready, or not yet ready to take action in the areas in which you are not currently thriving?

_____

_____

5. If you're ready to take action, I invite you to come up with three small steps you can take to enhance the areas of your wellness that need more loving attention.

_____

_____

_____

6. How would your life immediately change? How good would it feel?

_____

_____

Taking Action When You Don't Feel Like It

> " *The secret of getting ahead is getting started. The secret of getting started is breaking your complex overwhelming tasks into small manageable tasks, and then starting on the first one.* —Mark Twain

The most challenging aspect of living wellness is often taking action when you don't feel like it. No matter how committed you are there may be days when it feels like a monumental effort to get to the "starting line." On these days, it's likely limiting inner voices will do everything in their power to create internal resistance: *I have too much to do. I'm too tired. This will be boring. I can do it later. I should be doing ___.* Getting over the hump and taking action even if you don't want to is an important piece to staying consistent and connected for life.

An example of taking action is making food choices that are aligned with your intention and vision. Most of us spend way too much time pondering, obsessing, rationalizing, procrastinating, and debating action. This is a significant energy drain and makes choices seem more involved than they need to be. Maintaining your wellness connection is a result of less obsessing and more acting. Here are some suggested strategies for living well:

KEEP IT SIMPLE

If you feel overwhelmed, choose one aspect of your program to focus on. This will set you up for success by breaking your program down into small, "bite-size" pieces. For example, focus on drinking more water. Remember, there is no right way, only the way that feels right to you!

CREATE A HABIT

- Cook on the weekend and have your meals ready to go on Monday morning.
- If you're going out to eat, plan ahead. What kinds of foods will be available?
  Eat half the meal and take the other half home.
- Have a special water bottle for the car and commute.
- Designate a time to exercise. This is your time, an appointment with yourself.
  Guard your time fiercely.

BE PREPARED

- Pack your exercise bag the night before and put it in your car.
  Review your workout for the day.
- If you find yourself obsessing or procrastinating, have a power word or mantra
  ready to challenge inner gremlins. After you use your power mantra, take action,
  no matter how small! You'll be amazed at the power and momentum that's
  created by arguing with the limiting voices and taking charge.
- Take action now!
- This is my time. I deserve it!
- What is the next small step?

USE THE FIVE-MINUTE EXERCISE RULE

If you have no desire to exercise, tell yourself that if after five minutes you still feel the same way you can stop. Chances are you'll want to continue. If you still aren't into it, stop and resume the next day.

TAKE TEN MINDFUL BREATHS

If you're craving a food that is not an "optimal choice" in the present moment, take ten mindful breaths and ask yourself the following:

- Is there a better choice right now?
- Is there something "fun" I can eat that is in line with my intention?
- Am I consciously eating this or eating unconsciously?
- Am I feeding my emotions? How can I care for myself with something other than food?

STAY FLEXIBLE

If something isn't working, change your approach. For example, if you find it easy to blow off exercising after work, make the decision to do it first thing in the morning. If the cafeteria at work doesn't provide you with choices that support your intention and vision, go shopping and bring your food to work. Stay fluid. Adapt and adjust on the go.

BE CREATIVE

If you're on vacation and don't have access to a gym, do a Fit 'n Fifteen Express Circuit. If four workouts a week feels too overwhelming, cut back to three. You're in charge here. Remember, where there's a will, there's a way!

Daily Mindfulness

 The part can never be well unless the whole is well. — *Plato*

Life can get hectic and it's often hard to keep living well in the forefront of your mind. This can lead to mindless actions that contradict your intention, vision, and overall health. Have you ever done something and then asked yourself, "Why did I just do that?" Taking a few minutes during the day to emotionally anchor yourself to your intention and vision keeps you connected and assists you in making conscious, empowered choices.

Here are some suggested strategies for staying mindful:

MORNING AFFIRMATION

The moment you wake up, recite an empowering mantra. For example:

- Today I am committed to making choices that support my intention and vision. I intend and deserve to feel good now! I am deciding to have a fantastic day!
- I am in complete control of my thoughts, feelings, and actions today. No event or person can change that!

MORNING POWER QUESTIONS

Develop three Power Questions to ask yourself each morning before you get out of bed. The intention of each question is to put you in a positive, empowered state as you begin your day. Below are my top four power questions:

- What am I the most grateful for?
- What do I want to stand for today? Who do I intend to be?
- What can I do for myself today to support my intention to live well?
- What can I do for someone I care about today?

MORNING JUMP-START

Begin each day with two to thirty minutes of quiet contemplation. This can be done through meditation, while lying in bed, taking a mindful walk, etc. Dwell on all the grace in your life. Say a silent thank-you for a new day full of unlimited possibilities!

EVENING REFLECTION

Spend a few minutes reflecting on your day. I invite you to use the following questions as a guide:

- How was I successful today?
- What kind of challenges did I face today?
- How can I let go of thoughts and feelings associated with these challenges? Do I need to forgive someone? Do I need to apologize? Do I need to forgive myself?
- How can I learn from these challenges?
- What about my program is working? What needs adapting? Do I need to change my approach?
- Did I feel connected to my purpose today? Why or why not? Was living wellness a priority to me today? If not, how can I get more connected tomorrow?
- What am I most grateful for?

VISUAL/PHYSICAL ANCHORS

Keep something with you that anchors you to your intention and vision. For example, an inspiring picture, special rock, or bracelet. During the creation of this book, I placed a two-inch metal sculpture of a person (whom I named Bliss) next to my computer when I wrote and in my pocket when I wasn't writing. Bliss was with me every day as a constant reminder of my purpose and vision.

JOURNALING

In addition to cultivating your whole power provisions and documenting your fitness and nourishment choices, jotting down a few notes about your daily life experiences is a powerful way to stay mindful, anchored, and connected to your wellness.

Have Fun

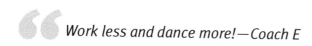 *Work less and dance more!—Coach E*

When your wellness choices become a way of life as opposed to a means to an end, you've made your connection! With this said, it won't happen overnight and if it hasn't happened yet, don't worry. It may take time to really enjoy your program, especially if you haven't liked to exercise in the past or feel as if your program limits you from experiencing other things you enjoy. It's hard to stay motivated and passionate when you feel as if your program is a burden or work. I invite you to embrace your program as an opportunity to be connected to the person you can and deserve to be! Remember, the purpose of dancing is not to get from one end of the dance floor to the other. Dancing is about freely expressing yourself through movement. Make your program a fitness and wellness dance. Keep it light and fun. Notice what feels good and makes you happy, and then do it! Here are some suggested strategies for keeping it light and fun:

MAKE IT FUN

Choose activities that you enjoy. For example, try power walking or dancing as your primary cardiovascular activity. It may feel challenging at first, but trust that your body will adapt to the new stimulus. It won't be this hard forever!

You may also want to turn your fitness program into a game. Set a baseline and see if you can top it from week to week. For example, include an extra interval or number of repetitions during your Power Circuit.

CALL ON YOUR POWER TEAM

Work out with a friend or member of your power team. This is a wonderful way to create mutual support, accountability, and time to connect.

FAKE IT

Pretend it's fun until it becomes fun! Play your favorite music when you train. Remind yourself how good it will feel after you've exercised or had a nutritious power meal. Keep in mind that everything counts. Every living well action (no matter how small) is a cause set in motion!

Make Yourself a Priority

If you're finding it challenging to follow through, it may be that your wellness is simply not a top priority right now. I invite you to make yourself a top priority. Your program requires energy. If your program is toward the bottom of your list of priorities, it's easier to put it aside or rationalize why "you will get to it later." If your inner block is around not having the energy for other important things or people, consider that you will have more to give when you pour energy into yourself first. How can you give away what you don't have? By taking care of yourself, you'll have more to give to the ones you love. SCIA creates an abundance of presence and energy that often spills over into every area of your life!

Get Some ZZZ'S

Your body transforms when you sleep. Cells and tissues are rejuvenated and your mind and body regroup from the stimulus of the day. Lack of sleep has been linked to illness, depression, irritability, poor focus, low energy, and decreased athletic performance. Often feeling as though you have no time or energy to exercise is related to lack of sleep. When you're rested, you have the emotional and physical endurance to make your program happen when things get busy. The take-home message is that adequate sleep is a vital component to health, fitness, and overall well-being. Here are some suggested strategies for getting more rest:

Make it a priority to get seven to eight hours of sleep per night. Some people need more, some people need less. I suggest using restfulness as a personal barometer.

- Keep your room dark.
- Do not eat a heavy meal within two hours of your bedtime. Doing so may inhibit you from sleeping soundly.
- Stop drinking caffeine eight hours before bed, or cut it out completely.

Your Turn

Contemplate the following questions and write whatever comes up for you without judgment:

1. **Have you made yourself a top priority today? Why or why not?**

   _____
   _____
   _____

2. **If not, what needs to happen for your program to be a top priority? How can you make this happen?**

   _____
   _____
   _____

3. **What would you be able to do with more physical and emotional energy? How will this transform your life?**

   _____
   _____
   _____

4. **Why do you need to make sleep a priority?**

   _____
   _____
   _____

5. **How can you get more sleep? What evening and/or morning activity can you cut back on to get 15 to 30 minutes more sleep?**

   _____
   _____
   _____
   _____

Liberate Yourself from Judgment

> ❝ *Health is a large word. It embraces not the body only, but the mind and spirit as well; . . . and not today's pain or pleasure alone, but the whole being and outlook of a man.* —James H. West

I encourage you to claim a guilt-free, failure-free, no-fault fitness and wellness lifestyle. Give yourself permission to be where you are at any moment without judgment, self-criticism, or guilt. Let go of the notion of "perfect" or "good and bad." Go with *your* flow, learn from setbacks, and have faith that your way will present itself. Instead of striving for perfection, consider being better than you used to be. Allow yourself room to evolve without pressure. Notice the inner space and lightness that's created when you decide not to weigh yourself down with expectations and "arrive" every day. If you fall off your path . . . be honest with yourself, let it go, and resume your quest! If you miss a week of exercise . . . let it go! If you binge on foods that are not in line with the person you intend to be . . . let it go and resume! If you feel as if you're constantly taking one step forward and two steps back . . . don't sweat it! The question is, how are you going to turn this "challenge" into a positive? The good news is you get to make thousands of choices each day. No matter how disconnected you may feel or how many setbacks you may have had, acting in line with your intention and vision will immediately reconnect you with your whole power. One action, no matter how small, toward your intention and vision immediately puts you back in the driver's seat. Stay open and don't give up! Here are some suggested strategies for liberating yourself from judgment:

BECOME AWARE

The light of awareness can overcome the worst of inner critics. Become aware of your inner critic by staying present. Be mindful of your thoughts and feelings. I encourage you to review your empowerment provisions, particularly Provision IV: Self-Care in Action, to help you silence your inner critic.

FIGHT BACK

Learn to argue with those limiting voices within. If you catch yourself in expectation, judgment, or guilt mode, I encourage you to fight back. For example, say, "This is a no-fault, judgment-free day. So, judgment and guilt, I have no time for you!"

Your Turn

Contemplate the following questions and write whatever comes up for you without judgment:

1. Do you allow yourself to "arrive" and feel complete every day, or do you load yourself up with feelings of inadequacy and guilt? How are these feelings serving you?

   _____

   _____

   _____

2. If you are weighed down by the desire to be "perfect" or "good," what needs to happen for you to let it go? How good would it feel to let it go?

   _____

   _____

   _____

3. When you have a setback, how can you immediately get back on track without mentally beating yourself up?

   _____

   _____

   _____

Actively Manage Stress and Anxiety

> " *The beginning of anxiety is the end of faith, and the beginning of true faith is the end of anxiety.* —George E. Mueller

We live in a go-go, do-more, never-enough society. Chronic stress and anxiety are detrimental to your health, well-being, and ability to stay connected to your intention and vision:

- Chronic stress and anxiety are risk factors for many health-related challenges such as depression and cardiovascular disease.
- When you're chronically stressed and anxious, your body releases a hormone called cortisol, which activates the fight-or-flight response. Cortisol slows down your metabolism and enhances the storage of body fat, particularly in the abdominal area.
- Stress can increase the desire to use food to cope with uncomfortable feelings.

- When you're stressed or anxious, SCIA often drops down on the priority list.
- Stress and anxiety can affect your ability to think, feel, and act in line with your intention and vision.

Here are some suggestions for managing stress and anxiety:

MOVE THROUGH STRESSFUL SITUATIONS

Stress is a physical and emotional reaction to internal thoughts or external events. The thought or event itself does not cause stress, but your perception of the thought or event dictates how stressed or anxious you become. The key to turning things around is knowing that there is little you can control in life, yet you can always control how you perceive and react to the situation. You're always in charge of your thoughts, feelings, and actions!

STAY POSITIVE

As you learned in Part I, positive energy creates positive situations. So ask yourself, *What can I learn from this situation? Am I speaking and thinking positively? Is my mind making this situation bigger than it really is? What's the worst thing that can happen? What do I have to be thankful for?*

FOCUS ON SOLUTIONS

Instead of dwelling on the "problem" and making it seem bigger than it really is, shift your energy toward the solution. What can you do right now? What can you control? Take a small step toward making the solution happen. Notice the momentum change.

DE-STRESS

Have stress busters in place so you can draw upon them during stressful situations. List ways to create emotional distance from the stress. For example, take a physical or mental break, if possible. Take a walk or mentally "unplug" for a while. Do five minutes of meditation. Perhaps the situation calls for "riding the stress wave" by being present to the stressful situation with faith that "this too shall pass." Decide to accept the things you cannot change and focus on the things you have power over—your thoughts, feelings, and actions. Work your empowerment provisions, particularly Provision III: Believe; Provision IV: Self-Care in Action; and Provision V: Positive Attitude.

Stress busters help you gain clarity, create inner space, and reduce the physical sensations of stress within your body. What stress busters can you use to alleviate anxiety related to stressful situations?

For many people it's hard to see the light at the end of the tunnel during stressful situations. The stress and anxiety seem all consuming and very real. Remember, you are not your limiting thoughts and feelings. Stress and anxiety are experienced within your body and escalate as you continue to feed the stress with more negative thoughts.

When you feel stress and anxiety building, take a few minutes to reconnect with your breath. Allow yourself to be fully present to the feelings within your body. Breathe acceptance and love into the parts of your body that are tense, and contemplate the following questions without judgment:

- What can I change in this stressful moment?
- What do I have to accept right now?
- What's the next positive step I can take to move through this stress and anxiety?
- Where else can I turn for help? Family, friends, mentor, universe?
- What needs to happen for me to let go of that of which I have no control?

GET ORGANIZED

Stress is often compounded when we think our day-to-day affairs are out of control and unmanageable. Give yourself time to get organized. For example, pay bills, return phone calls, run errands, or make appointments. Organization creates inner space and helps you regain control over your life.

DE-CLUTTER

De-cluttering your personal and professional environment is another way to create inner space, and physical space if you're training at home, to allow your program to flourish. Most of us don't realize the emotional toll a cluttered environment has on us. The physical act of organizing or letting go of clutter can be a cathartic purge of emotion that leaves you feeling light and energized.

TAKE CONTROL OF YOUR TIME

Break through procrastination by becoming a "doer." Notice how good it feels to execute and take care of business in all areas of your life. Delegate. Are there things you can delegate to others? Perhaps the grocery shopping, dishes, vacuuming, etc.?

Putting things off can subconsciously weigh you down and fuel anxiety. There may be times where living well means scaling back, taking on less, or setting boundaries. Stress and anxiety are usually related to overload. Keep things as simple as possible.

Your Turn

Take a few moments to contemplate the following questions:

1. What can you do today to regain control of your time?

    _____

    _____

    _____

2. In what ways can you simplify your life so you don't feel overwhelmed and anxious?
    What can you clear off your plate right now?

    _____

    _____

    _____

3. In what ways can you set better boundaries, take on less, or delegate?

    _____

    _____

    _____

Magnificent You

> *Character transforms, persona copes.*
> —*Kevin Cashman*

You're a magnificent original. When you take off your social mask and let go of who you think you "should" be, the light of your authentic self radiates. I invite you to let go of the notion that you are what you have, do, and look like. You are so much more. It is time to rediscover the "real you," the part of you that is more than just a body.

When you live authentically, you create the space and energy to follow through and evolve in your fitness and wellness life. Below are some suggested strategies for living authentically, letting go of negative energy, and injecting positive, healing energy into your life and the lives of others.

CLEAN SLATE

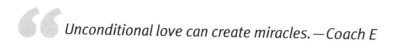 *Unconditional love can create miracles. —Coach E*

Decide to approach each life experience and interaction with a clean slate as if it were happening for the first time. Stay open to all possibilities by letting go of the past or what could, will, or should happen. Often we bring our history, beliefs, and anticipations to new interactions and experiences. This can cut us off from the limitless possibilities of right now. Imagine what it would feel like to be completely open in the moment to each experience or conversation without judgment or expectation. All interactions are exchanges of energy. Notice the charge you get from a mindful, authentic exchange with another person. Also notice the energy drain you feel when you interact with a person in a negative way. Notice how good it feels to project and surround yourself with positive energy. Notice the inner space that's created. Allow people to surprise you. Allow *you* to surprise you. You'll be amazed by the enriched quality of your relationships, as well as your ability to do things you once believed to be impossible.

Focus on Others

You only get what you want if you help enough other people get what they want. —Zig Ziglar

Taking a genuine interest in another person can be a transformative and miraculous experience—for both of you. It doesn't take much: a kind word, a thoughtful gesture, a moment of active listening. We all want to feel successful and cared about, and know that our life has meaning. The paradox is that receiving what we want is often a result of giving it away. As we discussed in Part I, the more you give, the more you get. So the take-home message is give, give, give! And serve, serve, serve! Help other people rediscover their greatness and your greatness will be fully revealed! Here are some suggested strategies for focusing on others:

LISTEN MORE, SPEAK LESS

During conversations, many of us are not truly hearing what the other person is saying. Often, we are just waiting for our next chance to speak. But in order to have a real exchange, we must listen, *really listen*, to what the other person is saying. The next time you are speaking with someone, remember to look them in the eye and show them you are fully present. Refrain from cutting them off to get your point across, and allow the other person to have the floor. A powerful energy is created when you let the other person know that you are fully engaged in the exchange.

Your Turn

Sit with a friend or loved one. Take turns talking for five to ten minutes about ideas, feelings, experiences, etc. When you're the listener, practice listening with your full attention. Resist the temptation to interrupt, interject, or teach. When you're the speaker, notice the urge to present yourself a certain way. Try speaking from an authentic place of not having to be anything other than who you are. How does this exercise make you feel? Take a few minutes to write down your thoughts.

_____

_____

_____

GIVE GENUINE PRAISE

Give compliments freely, expecting nothing in return. Focus on things other than appearance. *Appeal to the person's greatness.* For example, acknowledge a job well done or show admiration of a specific trait. Notice how the other person reacts. Notice how good it feels to give positive healing energy away.

SQUASH ARGUMENTS

Everyone has his or her own reality. Why is your reality the right one? Having to be right creates separation, animosity, and suffering for everyone involved. Why go there? Let the other person win—if it's so important to them. Notice how good it feels not to participate in arguments by taking control of how you feel and how you react. Let go of the need to win and be right. Ask yourself the question, "What was my part in all of this?" Talk about your feelings. Take the high road (if the situation calls for it) and feel the positive energy and inner space that's created.

LET GO OF JUDGMENT

One of our greatest fears is that we are being judged and, on a deeper level, will not be loved. As a defense mechanism, many of us point fingers and judge others—shifting the focus (and judgment) onto someone else. This behavior moves us away from being our best selves.

Perhaps the greatest gift you can give another person (and yourself) is unconditional love. Non-judgment heals and transforms. It gives us the freedom to connect with our greatness. Tell others through your actions and words that you are not judging them. This simple act can create miracles.

AVOID COMPARISONS

Instead of comparing and competing with other people, seek to consistently improve yourself. Turn the drive to be competitive inward. Do things that challenge and perhaps scare you every day. For example, strike up a conversation with a stranger, take a class in a subject that interests you, or enter your first 5K. Also, be on the lookout for people who embody living wellness and model them. See people as allies as opposed to adversaries. Both allies and adversaries can teach us what we need to know to move into our wholeness. Silently thank them for helping you strive to transcend your preconceived limitations.

SPEND TIME WITH LOVED ONES

> *The 'I' in illness is isolation, and the crucial letters in wellness are 'we.'—Unknown*

Spending time with people you care about and who care about you has invaluable benefits. Studies show that spending time with loved ones:

- strengthens the immune system, helping to prevent and heal illness
- combats anxiety and depression
- helps to build a support network for challenging times
- adds enjoyment and "color" to life

I encourage you to cultivate your current friendships and seek to reach out and build new ones. Also, take stock of your current relationships. Are they energy giving or energy taking? Are your friends supportive and encouraging or judgmental? I suggest you take a hard look at any negative relationships and consider letting them go. Have the courage to create the space for new, loving, and affirming relationships that speak to your heart. You deserve that. Have faith that the right relationships will show up.

For some people the challenge is creating the space to cultivate relationships. Often, other things in our lives take up a lot of energy at the cost of quality time with loved ones. While there's nothing wrong with caring about "things," evaluate what may be standing in the way of connecting with others.

Your Turn

Take a few moments to contemplate the following questions without judgment:

1. Do you focus more of your attention on personal relationships or on material things? Does your focus need adjusting for more balance? If so, how can you shift your attention to create more balance?

    _____

    _____

    _____

2. How can you enhance the quality of your relationships?

    _____

    _____

3. Are there any relationships in your life that drain your energy? If so, what do you have to do to let them go or, in the case of a family member, create the emotional space to radically take care of yourself?

    _____

    _____

    _____

Remembered Wellness

> " *Tug on anything at all and you'll find it connected to everything else in the universe.* —John Muir

One of the most amazing things about children is their ability to live in the present moment. To most children, the world is a wondrous place filled with unlimited possibilities and exciting adventures. I encourage you to think (and at times act) like a child. Choose to see the world from a place of wonder and awe. Nothing brings this point home more for me than being in nature. The natural world works in perfect harmony. Birth, life, and death meld into a miraculous and continuous circle of life. I invite you to spend time really taking in the natural world. Perhaps appreciate a tree blowing in the wind, sit by the sea, watch a bird fly through the sky, or hold an acorn in your hand. Know that you are a part of a system that's bigger than you.

It is important to remember that your core being is peaceful, harmonious, and balanced. In fact, we are all hardwired to feel good, to thrive, and to be well. As you've learned, the challenge is often that our thoughts, feelings, and actions disconnect us from our fundamental state of well-being. However, no matter how hard we consciously or unconsciously fight it, our mind consistently urges us back to this innate state. I call this coaxing remembered wellness. My hope is that the exercises, ideas, and suggestions in this workbook have inspired you to reconnect with your natural state of wellness and take consistent action toward the fit, vital, and empowered person you can and deserve to be.

Consider this the beginning of a new, ongoing relationship with yourself and the world. I want to thank you for giving me the opportunity to be your ally on this leg of your fitness and wellness journey.

I look forward to hearing about your personal breakthrough!

With gratitude,
Erik Hajer

Twenty years from now you will be more disappointed by the things you didn't do than by the ones you did do. So throw off the bowlines. Sail away from the safe harbor. Catch the trade winds in your sails. Explore. Dream. Discover. —Mark Twain

Let's continue to explore, dream, and discover together!
Join us at www.coacherik.com.

Acknowledgments

I could not have brought this project to fruition without the support, guidance, and love of a number of people.

It was my great fortune to be able to work with a group of brilliant editors and designers. To my editors, Carrie Grossman, Michelle McAuley, Emily Lawrence, and Jenica Nasworthy a heartfelt thank-you for turning my ideas and disjointed writing into a coherent workbook. Also, a special thanks to Sammy Yuen and Mike Rosamilia for their exceptional work on design and layout.

I am indebted to nutritionist Martha McKittrick, RD, CDN, CDE, for her expert consultation on Part III: Mindful Eating.

I am also deeply grateful for the endless support and guidance of my wife, Theresa, and friends Jonathan and Karen Roach. Your encouragement and unwavering belief in this project was invaluable.

In closing I would like to recognize my parents, Rob and Marilyn Hajer, who gave me the ultimate key to living my most fit, vital, and empowered life: unconditional love.

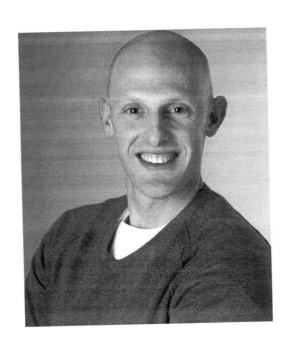

About the Author

Erik Hajer is an award-winning trainer and author who has helped thousands of people live the fit, vital, and empowered life they deserve.

Erik holds a degree in exercise physiology and was named one of the top trainers of 2011 by Boston.com. He is a self-described "wellness crusader" and avid athlete.

In addition to training "for life" he is a 12-time marathoner and 5-time Ironman Triathlon finisher.

Erik lives with his wife and two daughters outside of Boston.

For more about Erik and the Live Fit and Be Well Workbook please visit:
www.coacherik.com

Made in the USA
Lexington, KY
07 March 2012